Alcohol, Tobacco and Obesity

Although drinking, smoking and obesity have attracted social and moral condemnation to varying degrees for more than 200 years, over the past few decades they have come under intense attack from the field of public health as an 'unholy trinity' of lifestyle behaviours with apparently devastating medical, social and economic consequences. Indeed, we appear to be in the midst of an important historical moment in which policies and practices that would have been unthinkable a decade ago (e.g. outdoor smoking bans, incarcerating pregnant women for drinking alcohol and prohibiting restaurants from serving food to fat people) have become acceptable responses to the 'risks' that alcohol, tobacco and obesity are perceived to pose.

Hailing from Canada, Australia, the United Kingdom and the USA, and drawing on examples from all four countries, contributors interrogate the ways in which alcohol, tobacco and 'fat' have come to be constructed as 'problems' requiring intervention, and expose the social, cultural and political roots of the current public-health obsession with lifestyle.

No prior collection has set out to provide an in-depth examination of alcohol, tobacco and obesity through the comparative approach taken in this volume. This book therefore represents an invaluable and timely contribution to critical studies of public health, health inequities, health policy and the sociology of risk more broadly.

Kirsten Bell is a cultural and medical anthropologist and Research Associate in the Department of Anthropology at the University of British Columbia. Her research interests and publications to date have focused on tobacco, cancer, obesity, genital cutting and new religious movements.

Darlene McNaughton is a cultural and medical anthropologist in the School of Public Health at James Cook University, Australia. Her research interests include the nature of subalternity and stigma, the anthropology of biomedicine and the cultural dimensions of public health discourses on obesity.

Amy Salmon is a Clinical Assistant Professor in the School of Population and Public Health at the University of British Columbia and the Managing Director for the Canada Northwest FASD Research Network. She also holds research appointments at the Women's Health Research Institute and the Centre for Addictions Research of BC.

Routledge studies in public health

Alcohol, Tobacco and Obesity

Morality, mortality and the new public health

Edited by Kirsten Bell, Darlene McNaughton and Amy Salmon

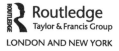

Routledge
Taylor & Francis Group

LONDON AND NEW YORK

First published 2011
by Routledge
2 Park Square, Milton Park, Abingdon, Oxon, OX14 4RN

Simultaneously published in the USA and Canada
by Routledge
711 Third Avenue, New York, NY 10017

Routledge is an imprint of the Taylor & Francis Group, an informa business

First issued in paperback 2012

British Library Cataloguing in Publication Data
A catalogue record for this book is available from the British Library

Library of Congress Cataloging in Publication Data
A catalog record for this book has been requested

ISBN: 978-0-415-59017-4 (hbk)
ISBN: 978-0-203-82215-9 (ebk)
ISBN: 978-0-415-82006-6 (pbk)

Typeset in Sabon
by Wearset Ltd, Boldon, Tyne and Wear

Contents

Figures

Contributors

Kirsten Bell is a Research Associate in the Department of Anthropology at the University of British Columbia in Canada. She has also held academic appointments in anthropology departments at the University of Northern Colorado in the USA and Macquarie University in Australia. Her main areas of research interest, activity and publication are: tobacco, obesity, cancer survivorship, genital cutting, research ethics and Korean religion.

Robin Bunton is a Professor of Sociology and has latterly been Director of the Community Evaluation and Research Unit in the Social Futures Institute at Teesside University in the United Kingdom. He has published widely in the field of sociology of health and illness with particular interests in: health promotion and public health, drug and alcohol use, social aspects of genetics and health governance and community interventions. He has been Editor of the international journal *Critical Public Health*.

John Coveney is Professor in the Discipline of Public Health, and Associate Dean in the School of Medicine, at Flinders University, Adelaide, South Australia. John has worked in clinical nutrition, and community and public health in Papua New Guinea, Australia and the UK. He has research interests in health promotion, food policy and food security, and has written and co-authored over 100 publications, including books, book chapters, articles and peer-reviewed papers.

Simone Dennis is a social anthropologist at the Australian National University whose teaching and research interests are characterized by a phenomenologically informed approach. She has brought this approach to bear in several contexts in publications including *Police Beat: The Emotional Power of Music* (2007), *Christmas Island: An Anthropological Study* (2008) and *For the Love of Lab Rats* (2010).

Michael Gard is an Associate Professor in Charles Sturt University's School of Human Movement Studies. With Jan Wright he is a co-author of *The Obesity Epidemic: Science, Morality and Ideology*, published by

Routledge in 2005. He has written widely about obesity for scholarly and mass-media audiences and is a regular media commentator on the subject in Australia and New Zealand. His latest book, *The End of the Obesity Epidemic*, was published by Routledge in 2010.

Rebecca J. Haines-Saah is a health sociologist and a postdoctoral fellow at the Centre for Nursing and Health Behaviour Research (NAHBR) at the University of British Columbia. With funding from the Social Sciences and Humanities Research Council of Canada and the Psychosocial Oncology Research Training Program, she is pursuing a programme of research that focuses on gender, youth substance use, and the visual culture of tobacco and drug prevention campaigns.

Helen Keane is a Senior Lecturer in Sociology and Gender Studies at the Australian National University. She has written widely on issues of substance use, addiction and health, including articles on medical models of addiction, harm reduction and human rights, compulsive sex, masculinity and anabolic steroid use, intoxication and pleasure and the uses of Ritalin. She is the author of *What's Wrong with Addiction?* (2002).

Kathleen LeBesco is Professor and Chair of Communication Arts at Marymount Manhattan College. She is the author of *Revolting Bodies? The Struggle to Redefine Fat Identity* (2004) and co-editor of *Bodies Out of Bounds: Fatness and Transgression* (2001), as well as *Edible Ideologies: Representing Food and Meaning* (2008). She is currently making a documentary film about the politics of the 'obesity epidemic'.

Lucy McCullough is completing her doctorate in counselling psychology at the University of British Columbia. She has worked as a research assistant and counsellor in the areas of mental health, substance use and tobacco since 2002. Her work in the area of tobacco has focused on evaluating the effectiveness of tobacco-control policies, health inequalities and the psychosocial determinants of tobacco use.

Darlene McNaughton is a cultural and medical anthropologist in the School of Public Health and Tropical Medicine at James Cook University in Australia. Her research interests include the nature of subalternity and the cultural underpinnings of bio-medicine and public-health discourses on obesity and vector-borne diseases. She is currently exploring lay knowledge of dengue fever in Australia and Vietnam and the social, political and ethical issues surrounding the implementation of new vector control strategies.

Michael Mair is Charles Booth lecturer in Sociology and Social Policy at the University of Liverpool in the UK. Michael's research interests lie in health, governmental practice and the sociology of scientific knowledge and his published work includes studies of tobacco use, tobacco control and the evaluation of particular public-health initiatives.

Svetlana Ristovski-Slijepcevic is a Research Associate in the Department of Sociology and the School of Population and Public Health at the University of British Columbia. Her broad research interests lie in the social and cultural aspects of health and illness. She has used perspectives from social theory to investigate how people of different ethnocultural groups in Canada engage with broader societal discourses about food, nutrition and health.

Robin Room is a Professor of Alcohol Policy Research at the School of Population Health of the University of Melbourne and the Director of the Centre for Alcohol Policy Research at Turning Point Alcohol and Drug Centre. He has worked on social, cultural and epidemiological studies of alcohol, drugs and gambling behaviour and problems, and studies of social responses to alcohol and drug problems and of the effects of policy changes. He has authored, co-authored or edited twenty-six books. Among his awards is the Jellinek Memorial Award for Alcohol Studies.

Amy Salmon is a Clinical Assistant Professor in the School of Population and Public Health at the University of British Columbia, and the Managing Director for the Canada Northwest FASD Research Network. She also leads the Substance Use Research Unit of the Women's Health Research Institute at BC Women's Hospital and Health Centre. Her research has focused on the gendered, racialized and class-specific dimensions of Foetal Alcohol Syndrome (FAS) prevention policies and on the health needs of substance-using women.

Preface and acknowledgements

Versions of the Introduction and Chapters 1–8, 11 and 14 were previously published in the Taylor & Francis journal *Critical Public Health* and have been reprinted with permission. The original reprinted material is:

Bell, K., Salmon, A. & McNaughton, D. (2011) Editorial: Alcohol, tobacco, obesity and the new public health. *Critical Public Health*, 21(1).

Mair, M. (2011) Deconstructing behavioural classifications: Tobacco control, 'professional vision' and the tobacco user as a site of governmental intervention. *Critical Public Health*, 21(2).

Room, R. (2011) Addiction and personal responsibility as solutions to the contradictions of neoliberal consumerism. *Critical Public Health*, 21(2).

LeBesco, K. (2011) Neoliberalism, public health, and the moral perils of fatness. *Critical Public Health*, 21(2).

Gard, M. (2011) Truth, belief and the cultural politics of obesity scholarship and public health policy. *Critical Public Health*, 21(1).

Bell, K. (2011) Legislating abjection? Secondhand smoke, tobacco control policy and the public's health. *Critical Public Health*, 21(1).

Bunton, R. & Coveney, J. (2011) Drugs' pleasures. *Critical Public Health*, 21(1).

Keane, H. (2009) Intoxication, harm and pleasure: An analysis of the Australian alcohol strategy. *Critical Public Health*, 19(2).

Dennis, S. (2011) Smoking causes creative responses: On state antismoking policy and resilient habits. *Critical Public Health*, 21(1).

McNaughton, D. (2011) From the womb to the tomb: Obesity and maternal responsibility. *Critical Public Health*, 21(2).

Salmon, A. (2011) Aboriginal mothering, FASD prevention and the contestations of neoliberal citizenship. *Critical Public Health*, 21(2).

This book emerged from a workshop held in the Department of Anthropology at the University of British Columbia in Vancouver, Canada, in July 2009 entitled *Alcohol, Tobacco and Obesity: Interrogating the New Public Health's 'Axis of Evil'*. Kirsten Bell, Darlene McNaughton and Amy Salmon co-organized the workshop with administrative assistance from Stephanie Gloyn. Funding for the workshop was provided by the Ethics Office of the Canadian Institutes of Health Research, the School of Public Health, Tropical Medicine and Rehabilitation Sciences at James Cook University in Australia, the British Columbia Mental Health and Addictions Research Network and the Department of Anthropology at the University of British Columbia, and we gratefully acknowledge their support.

Scholars writing in the areas of tobacco, alcohol and obesity from a variety of disciplinary perspectives were invited to attend the workshop. Most participants prepared papers that were distributed before the meeting and discussed in detail at the two-day workshop. In addition to the authors who contributed chapters to this book, participants at the workshop also included Peter Stearns, Rachel Eni, Leanne Joannise and Kieran O'Doherty. These individuals have made valuable contributions to the chapters contained here as discussants and critics, and we acknowledge their counsel.

A number of the chapters in this book, including a shortened version of the introduction, were initially published in a series of issues of the journal *Critical Public Health* in 2011 and we are grateful to the editors at *Critical Public Health* and Routledge for supporting dual publication. We are particularly grateful to Robin Bunton for all of his hard work in both suggesting and facilitating this arrangement. Finally, thanks to Grace McInnes, Melanie Fortmann-Brown, Amy Ekins and Carl Gillingham for their assistance in editing and production.

Kirsten Bell
Vancouver, Canada
Darlene McNaughton
Cairns, Australia
Amy Salmon
Vancouver, Canada

Introduction

Kirsten Bell, Darlene McNaughton and Amy Salmon

> Tobacco use is one of the biggest public health threats the world has ever faced.
>
> (World Health Organization 2010a)

> Obesity is one of today's most blatantly visible – yet most neglected – public health problems.... If immediate action is not taken, millions will suffer from an array of serious health disorders.
>
> (World Health Organization 2010b)

> Harmful use of alcohol has a major impact on public health. It is ranked as the fifth leading risk factor for premature death and disability in the world.
>
> (World Health Organization 2010c)

Although drinking, smoking and obesity have long been a focus of social and moral opprobrium, during the last two decades of the twentieth century they came under concerted attack from the field of knowledge and action that has come to be known as the new public health. '"Lose weight!" "Avoid fat!" "Stop smoking!" "Reduce alcohol intake!" "Get fit!"' is the rallying cry of the new public health (Petersen and Lupton 1997: ix). In many respects, alcohol, tobacco and obesity form the new public health's 'Axis of Evil' (to appropriate the rhetoric of George W. Bush) – an unholy triumvirate of 'lifestyle choices' deemed responsible for all manner of preventable chronic diseases, including three of the most common and costly: heart disease, cancer and diabetes.

Every day more evidence accumulates regarding the purported health effects of alcohol, tobacco and fat, and newspapers are crammed with alarmist reports outlining their devastating consequences. The tone of much of this coverage is judgemental. Headlines such as 'Drinking while pregnant risks autism in babies' (Templeton 2007: n.p.), 'Fatties cause global warming' (Jackson 2009: n.p.) and 'Secondhand smoke kills 600,000 a year' (Canwest News Service 2009: n.p.) detail the morally suspect nature of the smokers, drinkers and 'fatties' who 'endanger' themselves and others through their 'wanton disregard' for the unhealthy consequences of their behaviours.

One of the central objectives of this collection is to critically examine public-health policy and practice in the areas of alcohol, tobacco and obesity. Exploring this terrain, contributors interrogate the ways in which alcohol, tobacco and fat have come to be constructed as 'problems' requiring intervention, and some of the limitations of prevailing public-health wisdom regarding these three 'issues'. While it is not our intention to suggest that alcohol, tobacco and fat entail no negative consequences for health, the goal of this collection is to move beyond health (and in some cases 'against health'[1]) to recognize the social, cultural and political context in which public-health policy is conceived and carried out.

From causes to correlated risks: lifestyle and chronic disease

As Petersen and Lupton (1997) have noted, unlike the old public health, with its focus on controlling filth, odour and contagion, the new public health is characterized by an intense concern with the health status of populations. Although it has brought with it a heightened consciousness of risks that are believed to lie beyond the individual's control (e.g. pollution, global warming, etc.), it has also ushered in an increasing concern with individual responsibility, self-control and lifestyle.

Despite this marked shift in emphasis from infectious disease to individual lifestyle, conceptual frameworks underwriting the 'old' public health have fundamentally informed the professional vision of the 'new' public health (Inhorn and Whittle 2001). For example, although alcohol consumption, smoking and obesity are increasingly framed through the medicalized language of an 'epidemic' (see Mair and LeBesco's chapters in this volume), the 'dangers' they represent are vastly different from those associated with the epidemics of malaria, smallpox and cholera that wreaked havoc at the turn of the twentieth century (Brandt 1997). As Crawford (2006: 403) notes:

> Most contemporary dangers to health, unlike an approaching epidemic, are not immediately apparent. Disease or symptoms may not appear for years, even decades. Both the pervasiveness of dangers and their prolonged time-span require a medically informed, vigilant and sustained awareness.... Thus, to be health conscious today is to come into an understanding that one's health is in continuous jeopardy.

The transition from infectious to chronic diseases has thus brought with it a shift from tracking the singular 'cause' of disease to identifying 'risks': the social, environmental and behavioural variables statistically associated with patterns of chronic disease (Brandt 1997). In consequence, most chronic diseases are now viewed as a failure to take appropriate precautions against publicly identified risks – 'a failure of individual control, a lack of self-discipline, an intrinsic moral failing' (Brandt 1997: 64).

Present notions of health and disease privatize the struggle for generalized well-being (Crawford 1980). Indeed, privatized risk management is a fundamental expectation of citizens under the conditions of contemporary forms of neoliberal governance (Crawford 1980; Rose 1993, 1999; Petersen and Lupton 1997). For example, the influential health economist Victor Fuchs (1998: 4–5) has observed that, 'Every day in manifold ways (such as overeating or smoking) we make choices that affect our health, and it is clear we frequently place a higher value on satisfying other wants'. The answer, as Fuchs (1998) and others see it, is to encourage individuals to 'choose health'[2] via personal lifestyle modifications: to make 'rational' choices between healthcare needs and scarce resources.

Yet, despite the confident predictions by public-health officials and the popular media about the imminent medical, social and economic costs if the 'epidemic' of tobacco use, alcohol overconsumption and obesity is left unchecked, the impacts of alcohol, tobacco and fat are far from straightforward (e.g. Jackson 1994; Gostin 1997; Campos 2004; Gard and Wright 2005; Kloner and Rezkalla 2007; Walzem 2008). As Brandt (1997) has pointed out, the early epidemiological studies linking cigarette smoking with lung cancer fundamentally transformed notions of causality. The term 'cause' implies a single process in which A leads to B; however, the rise of epidemiology was accompanied by an emphasis on multiple causation in explaining the roots of disease (Krieger 1994; Brandt 1997).

Underlying multiple causation theories and the sophisticated techniques used to map them (e.g. computer-generated multivariance analyses) is a hidden reliance on a framework of biomedical individualism (Krieger 1994). As Brandt (1997: 67) notes, 'The irony is that the process of pathogenesis is so complex and overdetermined that discussion of "cause" necessarily becomes a socially constructed and often contested domain.' Paraphrasing Austin (1999), a central contention of this collection is that current assessments of the state of evidence regarding the health 'risks' attached to alcohol, tobacco and fat should be viewed as an ideological project as much as an empirically driven one.

Clean-living movements: the Victorian roots of the contemporary lifestyle crusade

Although we appear to be at a juncture in which lifestyle factors have acquired a unique prominence in public-health policy and practice, many of the contemporary claims about alcohol, tobacco and fat have historical precedence. Indeed, the Victorian era witnessed a sustained attack on all three substances that bears a striking resemblance to many of the claims made against them today (Engs 2001; see also Brandt 1997).

Temperance movements gained mass support in a number of countries in the nineteenth century, particularly amongst the middle classes (Aaron and Musto 1981; Gusfield 1986; Engs 2001). As is now well-documented, temperance reformers perceived alcohol as the root of social, moral and physical decay, linking it to familial violence, crime, poverty, insanity and a litany of other social evils (see Aaron and Musto 1981; Gusfield 1986; Levine 1993). At its height, the temperance movement was highly influential in countries such as the USA, the UK, Canada and Australia,[3] leading to a variety of alcohol restrictions and culminating in the USA's failed experiment with alcohol prohibition between 1920–1933.

The anti-tobacco movement similarly gained strength in the mid-to-late-nineteenth century. Like alcohol, tobacco was linked to various health issues, but of greater concern to social reformers was its association with the corruption of innocence and a host of other medico-moral issues that were the mainstay of Victorian medicine, including insanity, idleness, hysteria and impotence (Hilton and Nightingale 1998). Interestingly, smoking and drinking were often teamed together 'as an evil partnership threatening to undermine physical and moral health' (Aaron and Musto 1981: 176; see also Engs 2001). Thus, the UK and US anti-tobacco movements gained support from many of the same people who supported the temperance movement (Hilton and Nightingale 1998; Tate 1999; Engs 2001).

The history of the dieting movement also exhibits strong connections with the temperance movement. Many temperance leaders were also concerned with other so-called 'evils' such as gluttony (Schwartz 1986; Engs 2001); for example, Sylvester Graham was an American temperance lecturer who also became preoccupied with diet and lifestyle more broadly (Schwartz 1986; Engs 2001). The rise of 'Grahamism', where ardent followers pursued a healthy lifestyle through abstinence from alcohol and tobacco, restrictive vegetarian diets and regular exercise regimes, was notable for the way in which health reform was turned overtly into a moral crusade (Engs 2001; see also Warner 2009 for a discussion of evangelical Christian physiologists).

Clearly, although the strength of these three reform movements and the personnel involved differed across issues, temporal periods and locales, they were part of a larger Protestant-infused 'clean living' movement that ascribed moral value to self-restraint and self-regulation, and condemned 'pathological' excess (Engs 2001; Warner 2008; see also Coveney, this volume). Although the present public-health attacks on lifestyle are cloaked in the language of science rather than morality, they manifest considerable continuity with earlier claims. As Crawford (1980) points out, underlying the lifestyle emphasis of contemporary understandings of health is the assumption that what people are really suffering from is over-indulgence of the good society that must be checked.

Alcohol, tobacco and fat: convergences and divergences

Although alcohol, tobacco and fat have been a central focus of medico-moral crusades over the past two centuries, the historical and contemporary differences between these movements should not be elided. For example, for much of this period the anti-smoking movement was far smaller in membership and influence than the temperance and dieting movements, although it experienced a substantial reversal of fortunes in the mid-to-late-twentieth century as the epidemiological studies linking first smoking and then passive smoking with lung cancer emerged. Stearns (1997) argues that the turn-of-the-century campaign against fat differed greatly from the later wide-scale attack on smoking, despite their similar moral overtones, because medical evidence clearly set the stage for a transformation in public attitudes towards tobacco. Whereas, 'in the case of fat, Americans assimilated a new understanding that overweight could be a health risk that on the whole simply substantiated and justified a belief that had already taken root' (Stearns 1997: 25–26).

Another key difference was that tobacco use successfully escaped the 'rediscovery of addiction' (Levine 1978) that characterized attitudes towards alcohol in the early-to-mid-twentieth century. Indeed, the influence of addictions discourses was far more pronounced in the dieting movement during this period than in anti-smoking propaganda. For example, Esther Manz created the first national dieting association in the USA, 'Take Off Pounds Sensibly', after she was exposed to Alcoholics Anonymous (AA) messages, leading to her epiphany that her substance of choice was food rather than alcohol (Schwartz 1986: 25). AA provided a direct model for Overeaters Anonymous, founded in 1960, and the manifold other dieting organizations that followed, such as Weight Watchers, which has continued to retain a focus on public confession and mutual aid meetings integral to the AA model (Schwartz 1986: 204).

Tobacco resisted the realm of addiction for so long because the central defining feature of this concept as a cultural category is the idea that its use causes intoxication and behaviours that would not otherwise be manifested in the user (Room 2003; see also Keane 2002). Unlike recreational drugs such as alcohol, heroin or cocaine, tobacco's main advantage is its compatibility with the requirements of everyday life (Sullum 1998; Keane 2002).[4] As Berridge (1998) has shown, smoking therefore emerged as a policy issue through a different route from alcohol or other drugs – concerns came out of chest medicine, cancer and epidemiology rather than psychiatry.

Important differences between policy responses to alcohol and tobacco continue to exist. Today, the emphasis on austerity and self-restraint evident in temperance discourses on alcohol has been displaced by the perceived virtue inherent in moderate consumption and easy-going compliance (Aaron and Musto 1981; see also Room, this volume). Interestingly, this shift is also evident in the transition from 'dieting' to 'healthy eating' discourses since the 1990s (Chapman 1999), where the virtues of austerity and self-deprivation have been replaced by ideologies about the sensuous pleasures of beautifully presented 'gastroporn' foods made from natural ingredients and consumed in an unhurried (if restrained) way (see Probyn 2000). Conversely, the idea of moderate consumption is almost entirely missing from contemporary discourses on tobacco.[5] Nicotine is now often labelled 'more addictive than heroin' (Nicotine Anonymous 2010) and the concept of the 'social smoker' is now understood largely to be a transitional category rather than representing a sustainable relationship with tobacco over time (see McCullough, this volume).

Who's the baddest?

Clearly, the valuations placed on alcohol, tobacco and fat also differ substantially. As the WHO quotes at the beginning of this introduction suggest, in most circles tobacco presently holds the distinction of being considered the most dangerous substance in the new public health's 'Axis of Evil'. The tobacco industry's dubious victory as the number-one 'merchant of death' is satirized in the novel *Thank You For Smoking* when an argument breaks out between the central protagonist Nick, a tobacco lobbyist, and Polly, an alcohol lobbyist, about whose substance kills more people. As Nick says:

> Look, nothing personal, but tobacco generates a little more heat than alcohol.... I'll put my numbers against your numbers any day. My product puts away 475,000 deaths a year. That's 1,300 a day.... So how many alcohol related deaths a year? A hundred thousand, tops. Two hundred and seventy something a day. Well wow-ee.
>
> (Buckley 1995: 128)

Complicating alcohol's status as a public-health 'evil' is the so-called 'French Paradox' (Simini 2000): the reduced prevalence of coronary heart disease in countries where red wine is regularly consumed alongside of a diet high in saturated fats. Although the health benefits of moderate alcohol consumption remain contested (Hamajima *et al.* 2002; Koppes *et al.* 2005; Tolstrup *et al.* 2006; Saremi and Arora 2008), it has therefore been more difficult to condemn as an unhealthy poison than tobacco.

There are signs, however, that obesity is beginning to encroach upon tobacco's reign as the number-one 'killer'. Obesity, the popular press tells us, is the 'new tobacco'. A recent examination of media comparisons of obesity and tobacco (Rosen and Smith 2008) found that tobacco tends to be treated as an issue that has been successfully dealt with – a waning problem or a 'war that has already been won'. In contrast, obesity is portrayed both in the popular press and public-health circles as a growing concern poised to supplant tobacco use as the leading cause of preventable death. Notably, the economic costs of obesity are often highlighted – and described as likely to soon 'eclipse' the financial burden posed by smoking (Rosen and Smith 2008).

Significantly, tobacco control is increasingly being touted as a successful model for combating obesity (e.g. West 2007). In public-health circles the assumption seems to be that fatness (an embodied state) can be treated the same way as tobacco or alcohol consumption (embodied practices). Despite the existing critiques of the inputs/outputs model of obesity (e.g. Campos 2004; Gard and Wright 2005), evident in such approaches is a semantic slippage between obesity and overeating – with the latter used as a synonym for the former and implying a causal relationship between the two. Therefore, suggested public-health interventions include: the provision of information about how to avoid overeating, providing treatment for overeating, regulating certain types of foods (through price increases or restrictions on availability) and reducing the social acceptability of overeating or eating too much of particular kinds of food (West 2007; see LeBesco, this volume, for a critique).

Such approaches directly mirror established tobacco and alcohol controls, from 'sin' taxes to restrictions on how, when, where and to whom food may be marketed and distributed. West's (2007) call to reduce the social acceptability of overeating also parallels the tobacco 'denormalization' campaigns that have become a core feature of global tobacco control policy over the past decade. Here, stigma is endorsed as a legitimate public-health tool (see Bayer 2008; Bell *et al.* 2010).[6] In this respect, developments in tobacco and obesity policies appear to have learned few lessons from alcohol and other addictions, where it has been recognized that *de-stigmatizing* substance use is crucial for encouraging timely access to healthcare and improving health status, particularly among groups already experiencing multiple forms of disadvantage (see Bell *et al.* 2010).

Punitive responses and disproportionate impacts

The implementation of tobacco denormalization policies and similar proposals to stigmatize obesity speak to the increasingly aggressive nature of public-health policy relating to alcohol, tobacco and obesity. As we have previously documented (Bell *et al.* 2009), where there are deemed to be harms to children or foetuses, proposed legislation is particularly punitive. Thus, women who give birth to alcohol-exposed infants are increasingly being criminalized, doctors are being exhorted to report parents who smoke around their children as a form of child abuse and childhood obesity has been labelled an indicator of child neglect. In all three instances, this rhetoric of risk is mediated by, and reliant upon, historically rooted discourses that position women of colour and poor women as 'bad mothers', justifying the removal of children from their parents' care (Swift 1995).

Punitive public-health responses have also informed the framing of 'lifestyle issues' in primary care, where recent debates have emerged about whether smokers, drinkers and fat people deserve the same access to healthcare as other groups. Indeed, there are a growing number of instances in Canada, the USA, Australia and the UK of doctors choosing to withhold treatment from those who drink to excess, smoke and who are overweight (Hall 2005; Kohler and Righton 2006; ABC News 2007). Health professionals who have taken this stance highlight the 'self-inflicted' nature of mortality and morbidity associated with drinking, smoking and fat (Hall 2005), and the growing demands placed on healthcare systems where resources are already spread too thin (Kohler and Righton 2006). These developments speak to the pervasiveness of neoliberal discourses in public health, which disguise the unequal impacts of public-health policies and interventions across the population.

As Petersen and Lupton (1997) note, the enforcement of state-imposed health regulations tends to be exercised upon the most stigmatized and powerless groups, such as immigrants and the poor or dispossessed. For example, in the context of North American and Australian alcohol policy, it is the drinking patterns of the poor and indigenous peoples that are generally problematized – a pattern that has continued from the Gin Epidemic in eighteenth-century England (Warner 2002) to North American FASD prevention policies of the present (Salmon 2004; see also Salmon's and Keane's chapters in this volume). Similarly, obesity has increasingly been framed as a 'disease' of the poor and non-white, and people of colour and the poor bear the burden of public-health scrutiny (LeBesco 2004; see also LeBesco and McNaughton's chapters in this volume). The unequal distribution of public-health attention is even clearer in relation to smoking, which is today most prevalent amongst those on the lowest rungs of the social ladder (Bayer and Stuber 2006).

Accordingly, by positioning smoking, drinking and obesity as 'diseases of the will' (Valverde 1998) made manifest through overindulgence, hedonism, ignorance and excess, the new public health draws on tropes historically associated with the poor and racialized groups, while in turn valorizing moderation, restraint and responsibility (attributes most historically intertwined with white, Protestant, middle-class values) as fundamental to achieving goals of healthy living.

Overview of chapters

This collection attempts to bring together some of those who are currently studying alcohol, tobacco and obesity. It explores recent developments in public-health policy and practice in these three areas in comparative, international and interdisciplinary perspective. Several key questions have informed the conceptualization of the chapters in this volume. How are smokers, drinkers and fat people constructed as 'problem citizens' within relevancies of the new public health? Are smoking, drinking and fatness equally totalizing or abject? How and why do some substances become defined socially as inherently 'unsafe' or 'addictive' while others become so only in particular quantities and circumstances?

Part I deals with the way in which public-health research and policy are produced, focusing on the social, cultural and political context of scholarship and intervention. In the opening chapter, Michael Mair outlines the means through which the 'new public health' constructs its objects. Using tobacco as an example, Mair shows how contemporary tobacco-control research re-conceptualizes a complex social practice (cigarette smoking) as a non-rational behaviour amenable to forms of causal explanation loosely modelled on those found within the biological sciences.

This section continues with Kathleen LeBesco's examination of neoliberal governance as a means of conceptualizing the relationship between the state and the individual around issues of fatness. Illuminating the tensions between the injunctions to consume less and spend more, LeBesco discusses state efforts to enlist individual citizens in the 'war on obesity' and the more aggressive measures increasingly being implemented for those who 'fail' to self-police. Through this analysis, she illuminates the limitations of contemporary conceptions of obesity and the 'obesogenic environment' and their damaging consequences for those who dare to wear the proof of 'excessiveness' on their bodies.

Themes of excess and individual responsibility also run through Robin Room's examination of the contradictory exhortations of late-capitalist societies to promote both excessive consumption and personal restraint. Through an examination of conceptions of alcohol embedded in temperance ideologies, 'alcoholism' and the contemporary retreat from alcohol control, Room demonstrates the continuities between the contemporary emphasis on 'moderate drinking' and Puritan ideals, which simultaneously serve the interests of those promoting neoliberal free-market ideologies.

An attempt to crystallize underlying ideological conceptions is a core focus of Michael Gard's discussion of obesity scholarship. In this account, positioned as both an observer of and combatant in the 'obesity wars', Gard constructs an anatomy of the obesity controversy. Moving beyond standard representations of the two 'sides' of the debate, he provides a complex account of the disparate groups who comprise the obesity 'alarmists' and 'sceptics'. As his chapter convincingly demonstrates, in the context of debates about obesity, nothing could be more irrelevant than the 'truth' of fatness.

Kirsten Bell comes to a similar conclusion in her examination of research and policy on second-hand smoke. Exploring why this topic has been such a central focus in tobacco control and public health policy, she argues that the 'truth' of second-hand smoke is far less relevant than its cultural attributes as a liminal substance that dissolves the boundaries between bodies.

Part II of the book examines the ambivalent place of pleasure in public-health discourse on alcohol, tobacco and obesity. Central to the chapters in this section is an attempt to explicitly conceptualize and document the sensuous pleasures associated with embodied social practices such as drinking, smoking and eating, and to move beyond rationalist public-health accounts of consumption. Robin Bunton examines the ways in which pleasure is conceptualized and organized under the conditions of contemporary consumer capitalism. Using binge-drinking as an example, he turns his attention to pleasures deemed to be troubling from a public-health perspective via some reflections on the ambivalence and contradiction in contemporary consumer capitalism regarding the intoxicated body.

Helen Keane takes up further the topic of alcohol's pleasures through an explicit engagement with the typology of pleasures Bunton outlines in his chapter. Using the Australian National Alcohol Strategy as a case study, her analysis reveals the ways in which intoxication is reduced to its harms in public-health discourse, resulting in a radical disjuncture from the everyday experiences of drinkers, where intoxication is a form of bodily pleasure.

Writing from a phenomenological perspective, Simone Dennis outlines a similar disjuncture between public-health discourses on tobacco and smokers' experiences, particularly the centrality of sociality, corporeal connection and rupture that are central to the practices of smoking. She demonstrates the ways in which smokers resist the moralized dimensions of state efforts to regulate their bodies and the profoundly corporeal dimensions of smoking as an embodied practice. Lucy McCullough also highlights the intrinsic sociality of smoking, examining the ways in which contemporary tobacco-control policies have attempted to use the sociality of smoking *against* the smoker via social 'de-normalization' strategies. Her chapter considers smokers' responses to attempts to stigmatize this complex social practice – which often have the effect of reinforcing rather than reducing smoking as an embodied social practice and identity.

Finally, John Coveney explores the 'problem' of excess and its emergence as a central project in public health. Using examples drawn from public-health nutrition, he argues that there is currently an explicit and organized backlash against the so-called good life and the 'consumptogenic' environment it is seen to produce. Tracing the historical roots of our concern with unregulated pleasure, he demonstrates the ways in which contemporary discourses draw on centuries-old Christian values that abhor waste and hubris, and, in so doing, he highlights the pleasures that hunger itself entails.

Drawing on critical perspectives detailed in earlier chapters, Part III examines the groups being targeted in public-health discourses on alcohol, tobacco and obesity. It asks the question about who is being singled out as 'risky', 'unhealthy' or in need of intervention in policy and practice around the new public health's 'Axis of Evil'. As the chapters in this section reveal,

women's bodies in general – and mothers' bodies in particular – are especially singled out as key sites of risk production, although the effects of
such discourses appear to be strongly mediated by class and ethnicity.

Focusing on conception, pregnancy and reproduction, Darlene
McNaughton argues that, although the true impact of obesity on conception or the health of foetuses is unknown, core assumptions at the heart of
obesity science have been taken up uncritically in medical arenas. This has
created new opportunities for the surveillance, regulation and disciplining
of 'threatening' female bodies and the affirmation of certain moral, neoliberal ideas and values.

Drawing on research with Canadian families, Svetlana Ristovski-
Slijepcevic explores how mothers respond to nutritional discourses that
encourage them to monitor, assess, educate and discipline their children
with respect to eating and food choices. She simultaneously takes a critical
perspective on the lack of consideration given to the broader political,
social and historical dimensions of people's food choices.

Turning her attention to tobacco-control policy, Rebecca J. Haines-Saah
critically explores tobacco-control policy representations of female
smokers. Haines-Saah identifies a number of recurring tropes in these
images, in particular, the gendered symbolic violence of anti-tobacco messaging. Drawing on research with young female smokers, she examines
how representations of smoking as 'unfeminine' and 'unacceptable' are
reproduced and resisted in everyday practice and in women's narratives
about smoking.

The collection concludes with Amy Salmon's chapter on foetal alcohol
spectrum disorder (FASD). Drawing together many of the strands examined in this volume, Salmon's chapter provides a critique of some of the
more problematic undercurrents in FASD prevention initiatives, through
an analysis of how neoliberalist, anti-colonial and public-health agendas
are enacted by the state (directly and indirectly) on the bodies of Aboriginal women and their children.

In collecting the chapters in this volume, we have sought to locate contemporary public-health policy and practice within its broader social, cultural and political context, as well as highlight some of the more worrying
consequences of recent developments in the new public health and the
paths along which it is being currently pursued. In bringing together critical perspectives from a range of scholars, we aim to expose and flesh out
some of the fascinating convergences and divergences between the three
health issues under examination here.

Of course, there is much more to be said than could be produced in a
single text and there are a number of other areas that could have been pro-
ductively explored in this collection. First, in light of the emphasis on
sexual behaviour and drug use evident in the public-health crusade against
'lifestyle diseases', we might have conceptualized public-health policy in
terms of a 'Quintet' rather than an 'Axis' of Evil. Second, given the

growing focus on corporate culpability for lifestyle diseases, it might have
been useful to compare constructions of the alcohol, tobacco and fast-food
industries in public health and popular accounts. Given the burgeoning
number of lawsuits against these industries (especially the fast-food industry), future efforts would be well-served to explore how these fit with the
arguments advanced in many chapters in this collection about the neoliberal and individualist orientation of much public-health discourse.

Finally, although individual contributors are differently positioned in
terms of the degree to which they treat alcohol, tobacco and fat as problematic, the chapters in this volume take, to varying degrees, a social-
constructionist perspective on these topics. We feel that this approach
provides a necessary corrective to prevailing representations, helping to
expose the social, cultural, economic and political roots of contemporary
public-health discourses. However, we also recognize that social-
constructionist approaches may be accused of 'problem deflation' (Room
1983), and failing to engage with the biological impacts of alcohol,
tobacco and obesity on the human body. Thus, there are challenges that lie
ahead in terms of navigating a middle path that simultaneously recognizes
the moral, economic and political underpinnings of contemporary public-
health discourses on alcohol, tobacco and fat, whilst recognizing that they
can also present problems with real consequences for individuals and their
communities (Madsen 1983; Moffatt 2010). Our hope is that other scholars will choose to pick up where this volume leaves off and that the chapters contained in this anthology will spur further comparative research into
alcohol, tobacco and obesity (and their comrades in 'harm') and the ways
they have been taken up as social and medical issues, as well as examining
solutions to their problematic aspects that do not merely replicate the limitations of existing policies and practices.

Notes

1 *Against Health* is the name of a new anthology (Metzl and Kirkland 2010) that
   critically examines the moral assumptions underpinning the concept of health.
2 *Choosing Health* is the name of an influential white paper produced by the
   English Government (Department of Health 2004) that typifies this approach.
3 Harry Levine (1993) has argued that countries that developed large temperance
   cultures had two things in common: they were primarily Protestant and they had
   a cultural preference for drinking distilled liquor.
4 Of course, these features of tobacco are culturally and historically specific – a
   notable feature of tobacco use in South America was its use as an intoxicant to
   facilitate a bridge between the human and spirit worlds (Wilbert 1987).
5 Although it does emerge in representations of cigar smoking, where casual consumption is commonly depicted as a viable option, and sports and film stars are
   often photographed with celebratory cigars.
6 On the one hand, West notes that obesity is already highly stigmatized and so
   'there would be little point in focusing on this' (2007: 149). However, his call to
   reduce the social acceptability of overeating amounts to the same thing, given the
   cultural potency of obesity as a sign of excess (see LeBesco 2004, and this volume).

References

Aaron, P. and Musto, D. (1981) 'Temperance and prohibition in America: An overview', in M.H. Moore and D.R. Gerstein (eds) *Alcohol and Public Policy: Beyond the Shadow of Prohibition*, Washington, DC: National Academy Press, pp. 125–181.

ABC News (2007) 'Hospital restricts treatment for smokers, fat people', *ABC News*. Online, available at: http://abc.com.au/news/stories/2007/09/03/2022267. htm (accessed 28 September 2008).

Austin, S.B. (1999) 'Fat, loathing and public health: The complicity of science in a culture of disordered eating', *Culture, Medicine and Psychiatry*, 23: 245–268.

Bayer, R. (2008) 'Stigma and the ethics of public health: Not can we but should we', *Social Science and Medicine*, 67: 463–472.

Bayer, R. and Stuber, J. (2006) 'Tobacco control, stigma, and public health: Rethinking the relations', *American Journal of Public Health*, 96(1): 47–50.

Bell, K., McNaughton, D. and Salmon, A. (2009) 'Medicine, morality and mothering: Public health discourses on foetal alcohol exposure, smoking around children and childhood overnutrition', *Critical Public Health*, 19(2): 155–170.

Bell, K., Salmon, A., Bowers, M., Bell, J. and McCullough, L. (2010) 'Smoking, stigma and tobacco 'denormalization': Further reflections on the use of stigma as a public health tool', *Social Science and Medicine*, 70: 795–799.

Berridge, V. (1998) 'Science and policy: The case of postwar British smoking policy', in S. Lock, L.A. Reynolds and E.M. Tansey (eds) *Ashes to Ashes: The History of Smoking and Health*, Amsterdam: Rodopi, pp. 143–162.

Brandt, A.M. (1997) 'Behavior, disease, and health in the twentieth-century United States: The moral valence of individual risk', in A.M. Brandt and P. Rozin (eds) *Morality and Health: Interdisciplinary Perspectives*, London: Routledge, pp. 53–77.

Buckley, C. (1995) *Thank You for Smoking*, New York: Harper Perennial.

Campos, P. (2004) *The Obesity Myth: Why Our Obsession with Weight is Hazardous to Our Health*, London: Penguin.

Canwest News Service (2009) 'Secondhand smoke kills 600,000 a year', *Edmonton Journal*. Online, available at: www.edmontonjournal.com/health/healthy-living/ Quitting+smoking+could+halve+heart+deaths/2517555/Second+hand+smoke+ kills+year/2325410/story.html (accessed 29 March 2010).

Chapman, G.E. (1999) 'From "dieting" to "healthy eating": An exploration of shifting constructions of eating for weight control', in J. Sobal and D. Maurer (eds) *Interpreting Weight: The Social Management of Fatness and Thinness*, New York: Aldine de Gruyter, pp. 73–87.

Crawford, R. (1980) 'Healthism and the medicalization of everyday life', *International Journal of Health Services*, 10(3): 365–388.

Crawford, R. (2006) 'Health as a meaningful social practice', *Health: An Interdisciplinary Journal*, 10(4): 401–420.

Department of Health (2004) *Choosing Health: Making Healthy Choices Easier*, London: HM Government.

Engs, R.C. (2001) *Clean Living Movements: American Cycles of Health Reform*, Westport: Praeger Publishers.

Fuchs, V.R. (1998) *Who Shall Live? Health, Economics and Social Choice*, Singapore: World Scientific Publishing Company.

14   *K. Bell* et al.

Gard, M. and Wright, J. (2005) *The Obesity Epidemic: Science, Morality and Ideology*, London: Routledge.

Gostin, L. (1997) 'The legal regulation of smoking (and smokers): Public health or secular morality?', in A.M. Brandt and P. Rozin (eds) *Morality and Health: Interdisciplinary Perspectives*, Routledge: London, pp. 331–358.

Gusfield, J.R. (1986) *Symbolic Crusade: Status Politics and the American Temperance Movement*, Illinois: Illini Books.

Hall, C. (2005) 'NHS may not treat smokers, drinkers or obese', *Telegraph.co.uk*. Online, available at: www.telegraph.co.uk/news/uknews/1505050/NHS-may-not-treat-smokers-drinkers-or-obese.html (accessed 26 September 2008).

Hamajima, N., Hirose, K., Tajima, K. *et al.* (2002) 'Alcohol, tobacco, and breast cancer – collaborative reanalysis of individual data from 53 epidemiological studies, including 58,515 women with breast cancer and 95,067 women without the disease', *British Journal of Cancer*, 87: 1234–1245.

Hilton, M. and Nightingale, S. (1998) ' "A microbe of the devil's own make": Religion and science in the British anti-tobacco movement, 1853–1908', in S. Lock, L.A. Reynolds and E.M. Tansey (eds) *Ashes to Ashes: The History of Smoking and Health*, Amsterdam: Rodopi, pp. 41–63.

Inhorn, M.C. and Whittle, K.L. (2001) Feminism meets the 'new' epidemiologies: Toward an appraisal of antifeminist biases in epidemiological research on women's health, *Social Science and Medicine*, 53: 553–567.

Jackson, B. (2009) 'Fatties cause global warming', the *Sun*. Online, available at: www.thesun.co.uk/sol/homepage/news/article2387203.ece (accessed 29 March 2010).

Jackson, P.W. (1994) 'Passive smoking and ill health: Practice and process in the production of medical knowledge', *Sociology of Health and Illness*, 16(4): 423–447.

Keane, H. (2002) 'Smoking, addiction, and the making of time', in J.F. Brodie and M. Redfield (eds) *High Anxieties: Cultural Studies in Addiction*, Berkeley: University of California Press, pp. 119–133.

Kloner, R.A. and Rezkalla, S.H. (2007) 'To drink or not to drink? That is the question', *Circulation*, 116(11): 1306–1317.

Kohler, N. and Righton, B. (2006) 'Overeaters, smokers, and drinkers, the doctor won't see you now', *Macleans*, April 24: 34–39.

Koppes, L.L., Dekker, J.M., Hendriks, H.F., Bouter, L.M. and Heine, R.J. (2005) 'Moderate alcohol consumption lowers the risk of type 2 diabetes: A meta-analysis of prospective observational studies', *Diabetes Care*, 28: 719–725.

Krieger, N. (1994) 'Epidemiology and the web of causation: Has anyone seen the spider?', *Social Science and Medicine*, 39(7): 887–903.

LeBesco, K. (2004) *Revolting Bodies? The Struggle to Redefine Fat Identity*, Amherst: University of Massachusetts Press.

Levine, H.G. (1978) 'The discovery of addiction: Changing conceptions of habitual drunkenness in America', *Journal of Studies on Alcohol*, 15: 493–506.

Levine, H.G. (1993) 'Temperance cultures: Alcohol as a problem in Nordic and English-speaking cultures', in M. Lader, G. Edwards and D.C. Drummon (eds) *The Nature of Alcohol and Drug-Related Problems*, New York: Oxford University Press, pp. 16–36.

Madsen, W. (1983) 'Comment on R. Room's "Alcohol and ethnography: A case of problem deflation?" ' *Current Anthropology*, 25(2): 183.

Metzl, J. and Kirkland, A. (eds) (2010) *Against Health: How Health Became the New Morality*, New York: New York University Press, forthcoming.

Moffat, T. (2010) 'The "childhood obesity epidemic": Health crisis or social construction?' *Medical Anthropology Quarterly*, 24(1): 1–21.

Nicotine Anonymous (2010) 'Facing the fatal attraction', *Nicotine Anonymous*. Online, available at: www.nicotine-anonymous.org/pubs_content.php?pub_id=456 (accessed 29 March 2010).

Petersen, A. and Lupton, D. (1997) *The New Public Health: Health and Self in the Age of Risk*, United Kingdom: Sage Publications.

Probyn, E. (2000) *Carnal Appetites: FoodSexIdentities*, London: Routledge.

Room, R. (1983) 'Alcohol and ethnography: A case of problem deflation?' *Current Anthropology*, 25(2): 169–191.

Room, R. (2003) 'The cultural framing of addiction', *Janus Head*, 6(2): 221–234.

Rose, N. (1993) 'Government, authority and expertise in advanced liberalism', *Economy and Society*, 22(3): 283–299.

Rose, N.S. (1999) *Governing the Soul: The Shaping of the Private Self*, London: Free Association Books.

Rosen, R. and Smith, E.A. (2008) ' "Health" at any cost: Popular press comparison of the risks of obesity and tobacco use', paper presented at American Public Health Association Meetings, San Diego, CA.

Salmon, A. (2004) ' "It takes a community": Constructing Aboriginal mothers and children with FAS/FAE as objects of moral panic in/through a FAS/FAE prevention policy', *Journal of the Association for Research on Mothering*, 6(1): 112–123.

Saremi, A. and Arora, A. (2008) 'The cardiovascular implications of alcohol and red wine', *American Journal of Therapeutics*, 15(3): 265–277.

Schwartz, H. (1986) *Never Satisfied: A Cultural History of Diets, Fantasies and Fat*, New York: Doubleday.

Simini, B. (2000) 'Serge Renaud: From French paradox to Cretan miracle', *Lancet*, 355(9197): 48.

Stearns, P.N. (1997) *Fat History: Bodies and Beauty in the Modern West*, New York: New York University Press.

Sullum, J. (1998) *For Your Own Good: The Anti-Smoking Crusade and the Tyranny of Public Health*, New York: The Free Press.

Swift, K. (1995) *Manufacturing Bad Mothers: A Critical Perspective on Child Neglect*, Toronto: University of Toronto Press.

Tate, C. (1999) *Cigarette Wars: The Triumph of the Little White Slaver*, New York: Oxford University Press.

Templeton, S.-K. (2007) 'Drinking while pregnant risks autism in babies', *Times Online*. Online, available at: www.timesonline.co.uk/tol/life_and_style/health/article3602704.ece (accessed 29 March 2010).

Tolstrup, J., Jensen, M.K., Tjonneland, A., Overvad, K., Mukamal, K.J. and Gronbaek, M. (2006) 'Prospective study of alcohol drinking patterns and coronary heart disease in women and men', *British Medical Journal*, 332: 1244–1248.

Valverde, M. (1998) *Diseases of the Will: Alcohol and the Dilemmas of Freedom*, Cambridge: Cambridge University Press.

Walzem, R.L. (2008) 'Wine and alcohol: State of proofs and research needs', *Inflammopharmacology*, 16(6): 265–271.

Warner, J. (2002) *Craze: Gin and Debauchery in the Age of Reason*, London: Random House.

Warner, J. (2008) *The Day George Bush Stopped Drinking: Why Abstinence Matters to the Religious Right*, Toronto: McClelland and Stewart.

Warner, J. (2009) 'Temperance, alcohol, and the American evangelical: A reassessment', *Addiction*, 104: 1075–1084.

West, R. (2007) 'What lessons can be learned from tobacco control for combating the growing prevalence of obesity?', *Obesity Reviews*, 8 (Suppl. 1): 145–150.

Wilbert, J. (1987) *Tobacco and Shamanism in South America*, New Haven: Yale University Press.

World Health Organization (2010a) *Tobacco Key Facts*. Online, available at: www.who.int/topics/tobacco/facts/en/index.html (accessed 2 May 2010).

World Health Organization (2010b) *Controlling the Global Obesity Epidemic*. Online, available at: www.who.int/nutrition/topics/obesity/en/index.html (accessed 2 May 2010).

World Health Organization (2010c) *Is Harmful Use of Alcohol a Public Health Problem?* Online, available at: www.who.int/features/qa/66/en/index.html (accessed 2 May 2010).

Part I

The cultural politics of public health scholarship and policy

1 Deconstructing behavioural classifications

Tobacco control, 'professional vision' and the tobacco user as a site of governmental intervention

Michael Mair

Introduction

One of the hallmarks of the 'new public health' is a programmatic concern with the part played by human 'behaviours' in the aetiology of illness and disease. Tobacco (mis-)use, alcohol (mis-)use and the complex of factors implicated in obesity are among its most prominent concerns. As understandings of the extent of the causal role of these 'problem behaviours' in disease and illness processes have improved, pressure has grown to find ways of doing something about them, to devise new forms of public-health intervention best suited to the specific challenges that these particular behavioural loci pose. In light of the stress placed on the behavioural dimensions of health and illness, it is unsurprising that public-health programmes in each of these areas, despite their many differences, often share a common purpose and design, typically aiming at the ongoing regulation and control of the behaviours in question; 'prevention' where possible, 'containment', 'treatment' and 'modification' where not.

Although much of the conceptual framework has been carried over, in grappling with 'the behavioural sphere' and attempting to encompass it within its legitimate domain of inquiry, the new public health – epidemiology in particular – has had to stake out a territory, intellectually and practically, that extends far beyond that which its nineteenth- and early-twentieth-century predecessors were in a position to lay claim to. Its empirical targets, its central objects, have changed, as have the key questions asked about them. The priority of contemporary public health is not simply to isolate behavioural factors such as smoking, drinking or overeating, and to look at the ways in which they causally connect to specific forms of illness and disease. Although the underlying physiological mechanisms remain an ongoing research concern, the important development has been a general shift in focus to treating the behaviours themselves as epidemiological phenomena, the problem becoming how to develop ways of isolating *their* causal antecedents, the 'risk factors' which increase the likelihood that (groups of) individuals will 'contract' those behaviours and so expose themselves to otherwise avoidable forms of harm.

In taking the 'behavioural turn', in other words, public health has made its business the examination of what *makes* individuals behave in 'health-risking' ways, the systematic investigation of the complex chaining of inter-twined sequences of cause and effect that identifiably connect disease outcomes to a range of determinants, variously conceived (Mair and Kierans 2007). By embracing complex causality, by adapting the tech-niques of the social sciences, and by outsourcing the laborious technical task of matching pathogens to pathologies to research scientists in genetics, molecular biology and organic chemistry (Raymond 1989; Susser 1999), public-health epidemiologists have been able to leave the confines of the laboratory and move outside to survey, through the lens of behaviour, more and more aspects of the wider human world around them.

The goal in what follows is to explore some of the processes that have made this move possible, to critically examine how in practice the new public health goes about constructing its objects, here 'health-related behaviours', working them up in the particular ways that mark them out and give them their significance within its particular field of 'professional vision' (Goodwin 1994; Bowker and Star 2000). In an area of some com-plexity, I have found it helpful to focus in on simple, concrete examples in order to get a better sense of the sorts of processes and practices involved. Due to my background as a researcher within this particular sub-field and because I believe it usefully exemplifies what has been gained, what lost and what glossed over in making the 'behavioural turn', I have chosen to concentrate on tobacco use, more specifically, the mundane classificatory practices involved in the work of counting smokers.

Counting, classification and epidemiological practice: the case of tobacco control

While ubiquitous, counts are far from trivial (Cicourel 1964; Churchill 1966; Sudnow 1967; Sacks 1992; Bowker and Starr 2000; Martin and Lynch 2009). Quite the reverse; due to their simplicity, vernacular counting practices are powerful tools in all manner of ordinary and specialized set-tings. Within the pure and applied sciences, as the philosopher and histo-rian of science Ian Hacking reminds us, the business of representation, defining a problem, and the business of intervention, acting upon it, are intimately related (Hacking 1983). And, in particular fields of investigation, the development of standardized methods of counting are central to that relationship as they prepare the ground for the stable systems of quantifica-tion and measurement that both rely upon (Lynch 1993). This is no less true of public health than it is of experimental physics. The practising epi-demiologist, for instance, could not begin to get to work on a given health problem without methodical ways of charting that problem's distribution, by distinguishing cases and then tallying them according to type (Lynch 1985). As elementary constituents of wider forms of public health and epidemiological practice, counts can thus be seen as part of what enables the whole enterprise to get off the ground, allowing epidemiologists to locate and fix in place 'the objects of knowledge that become the insignia of the profession's craft, ... its special and distinctive domain of competence' (Goodwin 1994: 606).

Counting smokers is a case-in-point. By choosing to include, in the data they collected, counts based on whether the lung-cancer patients within their samples were smokers or not, clinician-epidemiologists, like Wynder and Graham in the US, and Doll and Bradford-Hill in the UK, were able to make the connection between smoking and lung cancer. Their capacity to 'see' where smoking fit into the aetiology of a particular disease was thus shaped by the taking of counts and the binary system of classification those counts proceeded from; 'being a smoker' becoming the figure that was eventually highlighted against the otherwise undifferentiated ground of the case histories they were analysing (see, for example, Doll 1998; Susser 1999; Thun 2005).[1] Graphic representations of the relationship these researchers uncovered, starkly unequivocal, continue to testify to the analytic power generated by organizing their results in terms of the cross-tabulations that the use of this simple device permitted (see Figure 1.1). Whether the first to discover the relationship or not, it was this group of studies published in the 1950s, classics of biostatistical analysis and causal modelling, that was to have a decisive influence on public health in the latter half of the twentieth century. These studies brought the dangers of tobacco use to the attention of the post-war publics in North America, Western Europe and subsequently beyond, providing a spur to further and increasingly sophisticated scientific work, and helping, in the long term, to galvanize a global tobacco-control movement which now claims them as its originary texts. That researchers have yet to find something that produces quite as clear-cut a depiction of the relationship between exposure to environmental tobacco smoke and its impacts on health perhaps provides some explanation as to why it continues to be a live issue (see Tonks 2003; and Bell, this volume).

Sixty years after the publication of those studies, counts of the number of smokers in a given population remain the basic source of raw data upon which responses to the problem of tobacco use are based. In that time, tobacco control, like other areas of public health, has become an increasingly data-intensive enterprise, and its sophisticated population surveillance and monitoring systems are reliant on the continuous flow of massive amounts of information from and through the local, national and international 'centres of calculation' that represent the key institutional relays in its global architecture (Latour 1987). Given this, it is unsurprising that the World Health Organization (WHO), which presided over the construction of that architecture and plays a crucial part in coordinating action on

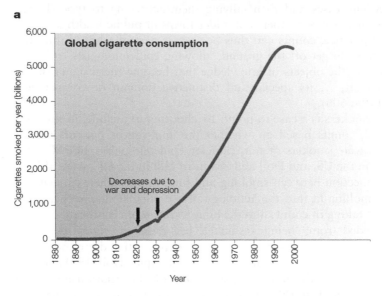

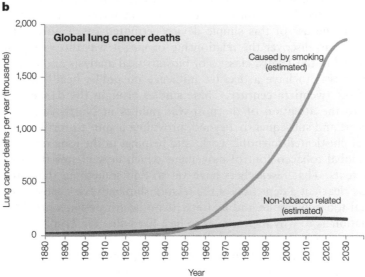

Figure 1.1 Tobacco consumption and global lung cancer deaths (reprinted with the permission of Nature Publishing Group).

tobacco control, emphasizes the importance of the collection of 'good' local counts, data which it regards as the essential building blocks of an accurate 'composite picture of the status of the tobacco pandemic in the early 21st century' (WHO 2003a). The WHO's landmark *Framework Convention on Tobacco Control*, which became one of the most widely assented treaties in UN history when it was passed into international law in 2005, includes a section that deals exclusively with 'scientific and technical cooperation and the communication of information' on the question of tobacco use (2003b: §VII). That section of the treaty, among other things, requires signatories to:

> establish, as appropriate, programmes for national, regional and global surveillance of the magnitude, patterns, determinants and consequences of tobacco consumption and exposure to tobacco smoke ... so that data are comparable and can be analysed at the regional and international levels.
>
> (WHO 2003b: 20.2)

Beyond publicly marking a foundational normative commitment to tobacco control, the extensive tables of information that are produced by these surveillance activities allow health officials to profile smokers in increasingly detailed ways, equipping them with a visualization device, an 'optic', that provides not only a view of the population as a whole but also the capacity to zoom in on particular 'at-risk' groups and deliver interventions in finely targeted ways. The biopolitical rationale that guides statistical surveillance of this kind, its general role in making populations manageable, has been examined by a number of celebrated researchers and social theorists, and requires little additional comment here (see Foucault 1975, 1998; Hacking 1990; Porter 1995; Scott 1998). What is worth initially emphasizing here, a specific instance will be discussed in more detail below, is the way in which this particular conception of research-as-counting ties directly into a particular logic of intervention. On the WHO's model, intervention, of which surveillance is an integral part, involves an open-ended commitment to further action (Hardt and Negri 2000). Although the problems it is addressed to may change over time, with crisis-management giving way to monitoring and prevention once problems are brought under control, ongoing action of some sort, appropriately modified to take account of the numbers, will always be necessary. Vigilance must be constantly maintained.

In relation to some problems – the great infectious diseases spring to mind – such a stance is clearly warranted. However, it becomes much more problematic, as is the case with tobacco use (not to mention alcohol use and obesity), when the 'disease' in question is no sort of disease at all but an activity linked to the way certain delineated categories of people live their lives (see Gard and Wright 2005). Here, intervention has a tendency to become highly intrusive, selective and discriminatory, and can serve to reinforce the marginalization of the already marginalized (see Salmon, this volume). When the same 'problem' populations are picked out time and time again, on behavioural grounds, for the purposes of intervention – indigenous peoples, the urban poor – they come to inhabit what Hardt and

Negri term, following Agamben, a de facto 'state of exception' in which they are partitioned off from the rest of 'healthy' society in terms of the differential treatment they receive (Hardt and Negri 2000: 17). Routinely re-describing activities that individuals engage in, like smoking or any other 'risk behaviour', using the language of the epidemic, has been one of the ways in which this partitioning has been practically achieved (LeBesco, this volume; Lavin and Russill 2010).

Behavioural epidemiology's practices of counting, exemplified in the WHO's programmatic ambitions for tobacco-control research, have, I would suggest, been central to recent shifts in the conception of public health's proper aims. The mundane work of counting smokers thus matters, and it matters for a range of reasons, providing, as it does, a means of mapping out particular kinds of problems, classifying particular populations and framing particular types of interventions. It contributes towards making tobacco use, and tobacco users, public, accountable and actionable concerns. There is, therefore, a great deal that we can learn by looking in detail at what that work involves.

As part of its drive to establish a global system for accurately measuring the spread of the 'tobacco pandemic', the WHO has encouraged the adoption of a universally standard method, examined below, based on a set of criteria that rigidly define what is to count as a smoker and how. The WHO's claim is that this system of quantification, which is able to weave together the local and the global in an apparently seamless web, is a neutral apparatus for 'carving the world at its joints', laying things out as they are in themselves before the gaze of dispassionate observers. However, establishing criteria about what is to count inevitably brings out some features of a phenomenon while excluding others, incorporating them within systems of relevancies that have important implications for the way in which it is possible to access and so think about the nature of the problems they are used to describe (Law and Lynch 1988; Goodwin 1994; Bowker and Starr 2000): numbers do not determine their own significance. Counting, in this sense, has a politics, what Martin and Lynch (2009), adapting Hacking, have termed a 'numero-politics'.

Once particular counting regimes are in place, however, it can be very difficult to work back from the finished product, the smoothly working calculative machinery, to the sets of assumptions and sense-making practices that give numbers their purchase on reality and imbue them with a moral and political import. Nonetheless, it is precisely at the points where particular ways of counting, and the representational schema built into them, have been most thoroughly naturalized that it is most important to subject them to critical scrutiny. As Talcott Parsons (1937: 10) has it:

> All empirically verifiable knowledge ... involves implicitly, if not explicitly, systematic theory [i.e. a body of interconnected propositions].... The importance of this statement lies in the fact that certain

persons who write on social subjects vehemently deny it. They say they state merely facts.... But the fact a person denies that they are theorizing is no reason for taking them at their word and failing to investigate what is involved in their statements. This is important since 'empiricism' in this sense has been a very common methodological position.... Marshall made a very apt statement apropos of this point: 'The most reckless and treacherous of all theorists are those who profess to let facts and figures speak for themselves'.

Taking heed of Parson's warning, in the following section I take a more detailed look at the way tobacco researchers get facts and figures about smoking to speak for themselves, to offer a preliminary sketch of the ways in which smokers are made available for the purposes of counting and to examine some of the problematic consequences of the techniques used to do so.

Behaviouralized description and the work of counting smokers

At first glance, counting smokers may seem to pose few difficulties. It is not, however, as straightforward as it might initially seem. Part of the difficulty is that smoking, as encountered in 'the wild', does not immediately lend itself to quantification. Until particular types of methodological decision have been made, the work of counting cannot proceed. This can be seen if we examine the example below, taken from the Liverpool Longitudinal Smoking Study (LLSS), which followed a single cohort of 250 children as they made their way through compulsory education (1995–2007) and used a mixture of qualitative and quantitative methods to gain insight into when and why some young people started smoking and others did not. In 2002, as part of the study, the participants were asked to write a short description of someone they remembered smoking. One girl, 'Lara',[2] wrote:

> When I think of smoking I automatically think of my dad. He didn't live with us so I only saw him a couple of times a year and every time I saw him he always had a lit cigarette in his hand and was always coughing. He died of lung cancer anyway probably due to always smoking and drinking. There's little I remember about him anyway because he was in prison most of the time but I remember him smoking an awful lot.

At thirteen, Lara, someone who lived in extremely difficult material and personal circumstances in one of the poorest neighbourhoods in the city of Liverpool, itself one of the poorest urban centres in the UK, was a heavy, every-day smoker who had started at a very young age, around ten years old. Unlike most other smokers her age, Lara tended to smoke alone.

The description Lara provides, while brief, is revealing. Viewed outside the context of a debate on tobacco research, the fact that the individual at its centre is a smoker would be unlikely to be the first or even one of the more salient aspects that someone presented with it would be struck by. Although a question about smoking supplied the cue, treating Lara's response as about smoking, rather than her father, would be quite misleading.

One of the things Lara's case highlights is that the sense in which she is a smoker is very different to the sense in which her father was a smoker. However, the sense in which Lara is a smoker is also very different to the sense in which those in her immediate peer group, i.e. young female 'social' smokers, could be thought of as being smokers (see McCullough, this volume). Looked at ordinarily, their cases are plainly not of a kind; there are all manner of differences between them. For Lara, her father and her peers, smoking acquires its meaning by virtue of its position within a particular setting, and in relation to particular biographies and relationships, making it difficult, because of the differences between these wider contexts of action and interaction, to see the individuals involved as doing the same thing, or to treat what is happening as instances of a single type of phenomenon. Even a truncated example such as this shows that smoking, far from being a simple 'behavioural occurrence' that can be easily separated off from its surroundings, lies flush with the activities it takes place alongside and contributes to.

One of the main achievements of the early studies into the health effects of tobacco was to effect a radical simplification of this complex area of situated human activity. As clinical epidemiologists investigating the causes of lung cancer, researchers had little need to worry about such things as the wider contexts of action and meaning in which smoking is embedded (see Bunton, this volume, for similar points on drugs more broadly). Context, a source of messy, 'thick' and often extraneous detail, could be bracketed at the start. Its inclusion would have impeded the investigation, making it more difficult to see, from an epidemiological perspective, the mechanisms that had resulted in the growth in lung cancer. Armed with the knowledge that it could be a factor, these epidemiologists had to 'thin' smoking down so that its effects could be systematically analysed in the same way as the other factors they were looking at, i.e. as a one-dimensional variable, either present or not (see Doll 1998).

Rather, therefore, than treat smoking as an activity connected in meaningful ways to others within a variety of overlapping 'forms of life' (Wittgenstein 1953), in a conceptual move that was to become the basis of standard epidemiological models in tobacco research and beyond (Crossley 2004: 236–237), these researchers foregrounded smoking, made it analysable, by operationally redefining it as exposure to a pathogenic source. For their investigative purposes, smoking did not have to be seen as either rational or irrational, but could be treated as non-rational, nothing more than an episodic series of specific 'exposure events', of variable frequency and intensity, in a sequence that spanned the given length of time from first exposure to last. The individual remained in this picture, just, but only as a shorthand way of referring to the biological system through which exposure was translated into pathological outcome, that to which exposure occurred. Apart from that, this definition makes few allowances for other distinctions and is essentially indifferent as to whether the 'individual' exhibiting that behaviour is a human, a chimpanzee or any other type of complex organism. Significantly, it is this definition that furnishes the four main criteria, i.e. type of exposure, frequency, intensity and time-span, that the WHO recommends should be used to count all smokers (outlined in Toque and Fullard 2004).

It is important to avoid stating in absolute terms that 'thick' description is always preferable to 'thin' (Ryle 1971). Crucially, however, the meaningfulness of thin constructs turns on the uses to which they are put. In a context of inquiry where the object is not people and their activities, but cancers and their causes, redefining smoking in the manner outlined above makes a great deal of sense. Nonetheless, while it is important to acknowledge the advantages of epidemiological constructs in some circumstances, we must also recognize their very real limitations in others. As epidemiology has switched from an examination of the causes of disease to an examination of the causes of the 'risk behaviours' implicated in disease, it has continued to rely on definitions such as that just outlined. The implications of this are troubling on a number of levels.

For one thing, in extending the logic of clinical reasoning, behavioural epidemiology operates on the assumption that analyses of what 'causes' an individual to smoke can be modelled on analyses of the causal relationship that connects exposure to tobacco smoke to lung cancer. The processes involved are treated as structurally analogous, making, for instance, 'having a parent who smokes' to 'starting smoking', what 'regular smoking' is to 'premature mortality'. We have no reason whatsoever to accept this analogy. Indeed, it looks stretched as soon as it is spelt out. Robust defences of this equivalence are, however, notable by their absence. Working within the 'disciplinary matrix' (Kuhn 1962) supplied by the behavioural paradigm of the new public health, tobacco researchers rarely subject the assumptions that underpin their own research practices to sustained critical scrutiny. The standard model is simply taken for granted as the only way of doing research of this kind. Indeed, it has actively worked to exclude other ways of thinking about the problems being addressed.

This process has political implications as well as conceptual ones. To demonstrate this I want to examine a representative case. The Centre for Public Health (CPH) in the UK is one of the new-style 'centres of calculation' that have emerged under the paradigm of the new public health. Like its counterparts around the UK, it specializes in the supply of 'health intelligence', the basic counts that make, as discussed above, more complex public-health activities, like tobacco control, possible. A huge ongoing concern, by the end of 2008 the centre employed 122 members of staff and still employs 84, the majority of whom are junior research assistants whose job it is to gather and process the massive amounts of survey data that represent the centre's main sources of revenue. Working to specification on strict turnaround times, these researchers are in no position to critically interrogate the applicability of the standard model to the problems they are analysing. It is not what they are paid to do. For them, the standard model is a 'black box' (Latour 1987), an off-the-shelf conceptual technology that can be used to transform answers on a survey into the descriptive statistics that are the centre's stock-in-trade. No special knowledge is required to process the information generated as the surveys anticipate their own analysis, making the task of working through them repetitive and mechanical. The primary products of the centre's routine survey work are self-published reports and press-releases rather than peer-reviewed journal articles. Opportunities for those outside the client–provider relationship to actually interrogate the claims made on the back of the centre's research activity are thus severely restricted. That what they do is shielded from both public and scientific scrutiny, and thus largely unaccountable, is a worrying development insofar as that work is often commissioned by policy-makers to identify populations for intervention.

In a recent publication, researchers at the centre analysed smoking behaviour among fifteen- and sixteen-year-old schoolchildren (Atkinson *et al.* 2009), based, tellingly, on data gathered by a private research consultancy on behalf of a governmental agency. They reported that, among those surveyed, smokers were more likely than non-smokers to: live in a deprived area; have more pocket-money; have parents who smoke; drink alcohol frequently, and binge-drink when they did; not participate in hobbies or sporting activities, or be a member of a club. The last on this list of 'risk factors' is of particular interest. In conjunction with the others, it is suggestive that smokers are anti-social, or perhaps more accurately, deviantly social, involved in morally questionable pursuits like smoking and drinking rather than healthy ones like hobbies and sport. The impression communicated is that these factors are attributes of individual smokers.

Yet membership of sporting facilities and youth clubs is a complex phenomenon. In the UK, research has repeatedly highlighted that having access to sporting facilities and youth clubs is a public good (Goldson *et al.* 2002; Davies 2005). However, they are also expensive to run and staff, and, if cuts are required, they are much more likely to be closed down before what are deemed to be more 'essential' front-line services. The region in which this research was conducted was one that had faced heavy cut-backs. As a result, there was evidence of growing inequalities in access, particularly among people living in deprived areas with a higher reliance on state provision.

Viewing the report's findings in the light of this information, what initially seemed to be a characteristic of individual smokers starts to look a great deal more like a reflection of the circumstances in which they live (making this an instance of what statisticians term the 'ecological fallacy'). Scrutiny shifts away from the individual and onto local-governmental actors. In this respect, the published analysis can be seen to have an in-built government bias. It absolves decision-makers of responsibility by deflecting attention from their involvement in the problem being reported on, while simultaneously providing them with a series of palatable policy options tailored to their preferences. After all, employing a smoking-cessation worker to go around schools on a monthly basis is a great deal less expensive than tackling the various forms of inequality and disadvan-tage that are exemplified by Lara's case (see Salmon, this volume, for similar points regarding FASD campaigns). In such situations, to adapt Foucault (1998), counting acts as a form of politics by other means, a highly specific process carried out by 'embedded experts' (Burnett and Whyte 2005) through which the tobacco user is constituted as a particular type of problem amenable to favoured types of response.

The underlying problem with extended uses of the standard model, examined above, is that context, the fact the individuals live together in a moral and political world, is systematically effaced by it (Herzfeld 2005). By employing the particular counting regime it promotes, the new public health cannot but treat individuals and not the situations in which they live as its fundamental problem. Its field of 'professional vision', shaped as it is by a narrow fixation on the behavioural and its causes, thus restricts the scope for open debate. For example, the idea, so obvious to public-health campaigners of the past, that issues like smoking, drinking and eating may be social, economic or political in character, and so require social, eco-nomic and political solutions, is simply ruled out a priori. That, I suggest, is a major cause for concern.

Conclusion

This chapter has been an attempt to trace how the new public health con-structs its objects by analysing the ways in which smokers are made to 'count' within tobacco-control research, a site of knowledge production where research and political agendas have become problematically entan-gled. Acknowledging those entanglements means recognizing the increas-ingly political character of research in this area, in terms of the kinds of claims being made, as well as who and what those claims are being made on behalf of. This is not just to repeat the truism that researchers have political views, or to note that their work can be taken up in unexpected ways by various political groups and actors (see Gard, this volume). It is, rather, to draw attention to the specific ways in which particular types of research, and research outfits, have become co-extensive with the political administration of public health, with researchers repositioned as numero-political agents helping governmental actors to bypass collective processes of deliberation by invoking the neutral authority of 'expert' evidence in support of the actions they take. Puncturing those claims should be an urgent priority. One area where deconstructive efforts can be most useful, in this regard, is in picking apart the assumptions embodied in the 'simple' act of counting.

Notes

1 The question of what 'counts' as the first scientific evidence of the link between tobacco use and lung cancer has been the subject of recent controversy. As has now been established, clinical epidemiologists from the 1920s, many working for the Weimar and Nazi regimes in Germany, had reached similar, though less rigorously evidenced, conclusions (for commentaries see Smith *et al.* 1994; Proctor 1997; Smith 2005; for a 'corrected' timeline of discovery, see Proctor 2001).
2 The participant's name has been altered.

References

Atkinson, A., Bellis, M., Hughes, K., Hughes, S. and Smallthwaite, L. (2009) *Smoking Behaviour in North West Schoolchildren: A Study of Fifteen and Sixteen Year Olds*, Liverpool: Centre for Public Health.

Bowker, G. and Starr, S.L. (2000) *Sorting Things Out: Classification and its Consequences*, Cambridge, MA: MIT Press.

Burnett, J. and Whyte, D. (2005) 'Embedded expertise and the new terrorism', *Journal for Crime, Conflict and the Media*, 1(4): 1–18.

Churchill, L. (1966) 'Notes on everyday quantitative practices', paper presented at American Sociological Association Meetings, Miami, Florida.

Cicourel, A.V. (1964) *Method and Measurement in Sociology*, New York: Free Press.

Crossley, N. (2004) 'Fat is a sociological issue: Obesity rates in late modern, "body conscious" societies', *Social Theory and Health*, 2(3): 222–253.

Davies, B. (2005) 'Youth work: A manifesto for our times', *Youth and Policy*, 88: 5–28.

Doll, R. (1998) 'The first reports on smoking and lung cancer', in S. Lock, L. Reynolds and E.M. Tansey (eds) *Ashes to Ashes: The History of Smoking and Health*, London: Clio Medica, pp. 130–142.

Foucault, M. (1975) *Discipline and Punish: the Birth of the Prison*, trans. A. Sheridan, London: Penguin.

Foucault, M. (1998) *The Will to Knowledge: The History of Sexuality*, vol. 1, trans. R. Hurley, London: Penguin.

Gard, M. and Wright, J. (2005) *The Obesity Epidemic: Science, Morality and Ideology*, London: Routledge.

Goldson, B., Lavalette, M. and McKechnie, J. (eds) (2002) *Children, Welfare and the State*, London: Sage.

Goodwin, C. (1994) 'Professional vision', *American Anthropologist*, 96(3): 606–633.

Hacking, I. (1983) *Representing and Intervening: Introductory Topics in the Philosophy of Natural Science*, Cambridge: Cambridge University Press.

Hacking, I. (1990) *The Taming of Chance*, Cambridge: Cambridge University Press.

Hardt, M. and Negri, A. (2000) *Empire*, Cambridge, MA: Harvard University Press.

Herzfeld, M. (2005) 'Political optics and the occlusion of intimate knowledge', *American Anthropologist*, 107(3): 369–376.

Kuhn, T.S. (1962) *The Structure of Scientific Revolutions*, Chicago: Chicago University Press.

Latour, B. (1987) *Science in Action: How to Follow Scientists and Engineers through Society*, Cambridge, MA: Harvard University Press.

Lavin, C. and Russill, C. (2010) 'The ideology of the epidemic', *New Political Science*, 32(1): 65–82.

Law, J. and Lynch, M. (1988) 'Lists, field guides, and the descriptive organization of seeing: Birdwatching as an exemplary observational activity', *Human Studies*, 11(2/3): 271–303.

Lynch, M. (1985) 'Discipline and the material form of images: an analysis of scientific visibility', *Social Studies of Science*, 15(1): 37–66.

Lynch, M. (1993) *Scientific Practice and Ordinary Action: Ethnomethodology and Social Studies of Science*, Cambridge: Cambridge University Press.

Mair, M. and Kierans, C. (2007) 'Critical reflections on the field of tobacco research: The role of tobacco control in defining the tobacco research agenda', *Critical Public Health*, 17(2): 103–112.

Martin, A. and Lynch, M. (2009) 'Counting things and people: The practices and politics of counting', *Social Problems*, 56(2): 243–266.

Parsons, T. (1937) *The Structure of Social Action*, New York: McGraw-Hill.

Porter, T.M. (1995) *Trust in Numbers: The Pursuit of Objectivity in Science and Public Life*, Princeton: Princeton University Press.

Proctor, R.N. (1997) 'The Nazi war on tobacco: Ideology, evidence, and possible cancer consequences', *Bulletin of the History of Medicine*, 71(3): 435–488.

Proctor, R.N. (2001) 'Tobacco and the global lung cancer epidemic', *Nature Reviews Cancer*, 1: 82–86.

Raymond, J.S. (1989) 'Behavioral epidemiology: The science of health promotion', *Health Promotion*, 4(4): 281–286.

Ryle, G. (1971) *Collected Papers, Volume 2: Collected Essays, 1929–1968*, London: Hutchinson.

Sacks, H. (1992) *Lectures on Conversation: Volumes I and II*, edited by G. Jefferson, Oxford: Blackwell.

Scott, J. (1998) *Seeing Like a State: How Some Schemes to Improve the Human Condition Have Failed*, New Haven: Yale University Press.

Smith, G.D. (2005) 'The first reports on smoking and lung cancer – why are they consistently ignored?', *Bulletin of the World Health Organization*, 83(10): 799–800.

Smith, G.D., Strobele, S.A. and Egger, M. (1994) 'Smoking and health promotion in Nazi Germany', *Journal of Epidemiology and Community Health*, 48: 220–223.

Sudnow, D. (1967) 'Counting deaths', in R. Turner (ed.) *Ethnomethodology*, Harmondsworth: Penguin, pp. 102–108.

Susser, M. (1999) 'Should the epidemiologist be a social scientist or a molecular biologist?', *International Journal of Epidemiology*, 28(5): 1019–1022.

Thun, M. (2005) 'When truth is unwelcome: The first reports on smoking and lung cancer', *Bulletin of the World Health Organization*, 83(2): 144–145.

Tonks, A. (2003) 'Summary of rapid responses to editorial: Effect of passive smoking on health', *British Medical Journal*, 327: 505–506.

Toque, K. and Fullard, B. (2004) 'Recommended standards for identifying smoking prevalence from local lifestyle surveys', *Centre for Public Health: Tobacco Control Research Bulletin*, 2.

Wittgenstein, L. (1953) *Philosophical Investigations*, edited by G.E.M. Anscombe, Oxford: Blackwell.

World Health Organization (2003a) *Tobacco Control Country Profiles*, 2nd edn, Geneva: WHO.

World Health Organization (2003b) *The Framework Convention on Tobacco Control*, Geneva: WHO.

2 Neoliberalism, public health and the moral perils of fatness

Kathleen LeBesco

Introduction

In late May 2009, I sat at my computer to begin drafting this chapter; a news alert popped up in one of my emails – a link to Fox News Carolina website. I clicked through to read the headline, 'Missing 555-Pound Teen Found In Maryland; Mother Faces Charge In SC' (Fox Carolina 2009). Accused of medical neglect, Jerri Gray, the mother of Alexander Draper, had fled the state with her son rather than face a court date in which her custody of him might have been undermined by the state. Their unsmiling, fleshy African American faces peered out from dark backgrounds in grainy, unflattering pictures just off to the side of the article.

Right smack dab in the middle of this news story was a large, enticing ad for the chain restaurant Wendy's: colourful, succulent, crispy pieces of chicken coated in a savoury glaze nestled on a platter, beckoning the reader. The copy, in bright letters emblazoned above the chicken, reassured us: 'It's waaaay better than fast food.™ It's Wendy's.' The healthy, vibrant consumer is hailed as *this* food is positioned as superior to the grub of the masses.

I notice and call out this juxtaposition not as a pundit lamenting the decline of American civilization – this is not a glib indictment of a 'schizophrenic' society that sells us unhealthy fast food with gastroporn imagery at the same time that it polices those who appear to indulge regularly in such decadence – but rather as a way in to thinking about the relationship between the state and the individual around issues of fatness in the context of a culture that is deeply anxious about consumption. This cultural demand for excessive consumption and chagrin at those who dare wear the proof of excessiveness on their bodies is evidenced at a number of sites (LeBesco 2004), but in this chapter I am most interested in how it plays out in the public-health establishment and the public imaginary about health.

Obesity and the good citizen

In February 2008, the Georgia State Senate passed a bill mandating that schoolchildren be weighed twice per year by school staff (Senate Bill 506, later lost in the State House of Representatives – see Georgia General Assembly 2008). The bill, which requires regular offerings of physical education classes as well as the posting of aggregate data on body mass index (BMI) on publicly accessible websites, joins dozens of other instances of legislation in the US designed to responsibilize the citizenry in the context of a great deal of panic about fatness.[1] In the same year, the Mississippi legislature introduced a bill (later shot down) that would have prohibited certain food establishments from serving food to fat people, based on State Health Department criteria (Mississippi Legislature 2008). Such efforts to legislate consumption and comportment exist not only in so-called 'fat states' like Georgia and Arkansas (the site of the first BMI bill), but also in municipalities with a sleeker image: New York City sends home 'fitness-grams' (NYC Department of Education 2006) and Philadelphia delivers 'obesity report cards' to parents of its schoolchildren as well (Hahnemann University Hospital 2008). These are not isolated moments of anti-fat anxiety; instead, they are part of a larger cultural landscape in which the state goes so far as to forcibly remove fat children from their parents' care (citing merely the children's fatness as evidence of abuse or medical neglect, as in the case of Anthony Draper), all in the name of health. Interestingly, much legislation that reeks of 'nanny-statism' for the general public (like the aforementioned restaurant bill) fails to be passed into law (Share and Strain 2008) and is vehemently rejected by those on the far right of the political spectrum (see Gard, this volume) – but legislation that targets the welfare of children is a much easier sell because of what we believe their health reveals about 'the permissive nature of parenting and potential moral social decay' (Coveney 2008: 199; see also Bell *et al.* 2009).

Public-health strategies in earlier decades tended to focus on public hygiene issues. Today, in contrast, the behaviour and appearance of individual bodies is far more important. The healthy body has come to signify the morally worthy citizen – one who exercises discipline over his or her own body, extends the reach of the state and shares the burden of governance. This chapter examines attempts by the state – via BMI bills, obesity report cards, curtailment of custody, and more – to enlist individual citizens in the war on obesity as they rehearse a reductive collapse between weight and health that may actually undermine human wellness. The chapter considers such efforts to responsibilize the individual citizen in light of recent arguments by concerned scholars (Critser 2003; Yancey *et al.* 2006; Berlant 2007) that the collective citizenry must revolt against the oppressiveness of our so-called 'obesogenic environment' if we are to preserve our good health.

Fat = unhealthy = bad

There have always been fat people, but the nomenclature of the 'obesity epidemic' is a relatively recent phenomenon (Gard and Wright 2005). A search for the phrase 'obesity epidemic' in the general news of major newspapers in English-speaking countries shows an explosion of interest, from just one hit in 1993 to 770 hits in 2004 (see Saguy and Riley 2005, for additional statistics). As Harvey Levenstein notes:

> Calling such things as rising rates of obesity 'epidemics' could be seen as part of the twentieth-century trend toward medicalizing ailments that had previously been seen as the result of moral failings – the kind of process that changed madness into mental illness and drunkenness into alcoholism.
>
> (Levenstein 2003: 262; see also Mair, this volume)

The manner in which 'obese, overweight, or fat' is collapsed into 'unhealthy' is unabashedly ideological (Campos 2004; Gard and Wright 2005; Campos *et al.* 2006). Charlene Elliott maintains that 'the figurative concept of citizen "fitness" is often mistakenly conflated with the visible look of leanness' (2007: 134; see also Jutel 2005; Murray 2005). Drawing on De Tocqueville circa 1840, she notes that active, working, non-slothful bodies are thought to be contributors to democracy, while the opposite are drains and detriments (Elliott 2007: 136). When we shift to an information economy in which physical strength is less important, the fat body is reframed as a drain on healthcare because fat people make bad personal consumption choices.

Such a shift in thinking about fatness is concomitant with the move to a neoliberal form of governmentality described by Michel Foucault (1975). Foucault sees us as normalizing certain kinds of bodies and making docile, obedient subjects 'voluntarily' work to approximate these norms under a gaze that keeps deviance under surveillance. Individual needs and desires are thrown over by a state that responds only at the level of the population:

> Population statistics identify a new form of deviance, the obese body, that endangers the welfare of society. Individual citizens are now asked to locate themselves within the BMI scale, to confess being fat and to seek the appropriate bodily discipline (diet and exercise) to avoid becoming an economic burden for society.
>
> (Markula 2008: n.p.; see also Petersen 2003)

In Foucault's view (1991: 11), practices of the self are not invented by subjects themselves but rather are 'proposed, suggested and imposed' on them by one's culture, society and social group (see also Whyte 2009). As the reach of the state is extended (but not by force), good citizens become partners in the governance of their own affairs and their own bodies.

Those active citizens who can effectively manage their own risk are starkly contrasted with marginal populations who require intervention in a manner that allows us to see risks associated with obesity as aimed at 'reinscribing and recoding earlier languages of stratification, disadvantage, and marginalization' (Dean 1999: 167). The intense focus on control of one's own body comes with a blind spot, though: there is far less notice of whether that control requires a lot of expense and less-than-healthy manoeuvres, as in the case of the bulimic, the tanning-hut habitué or the plastic surgery addict (Bacchi and Beasley 2002: 348) to gain a 'healthy' appearance. Fatness seems to equate instantaneously with unhealthiness, and thinness with healthiness, based on a false presumption about the transparency of these bodies in terms of the actions they undertake (LeBesco 2004). However, as Elliott (2007) notes, since we now promote indulgent routes to leanness (like the Atkins Diet), the fat body cannot be understood solely to be morally lax. As Elliot explains, 'The problem is not really moral at all. The real problem seems to exist in the conspicuousness of the body itself' (Elliott 2007: 143). The hypervisibility of fat bodies, then, triggers (often incorrect) assumptions about the extent to which fat people are appropriately self-governing.

As we think about these transformations in the production of citizenship, we must also think about how public health is implicated. According to Petersen (2003: 194), 'citizens are increasingly expected, as a condition of access to health care services, to play their role in minimising their contribution to health care costs by becoming more responsible health care "consumers", and adopting appropriate practices of prevention'. Health-insurance companies, for instance, have taken to sending out sunny, empowering, helpful brochures about prevention – ostensibly benign educational material that encourages the insured to adopt healthy lifestyles such as maintaining a healthy weight as well as blood sugar and cholesterol levels, not smoking, and so on. They dutifully instruct about what those healthy levels (always quantifiable) are, and highlight the bargain of preventive care as opposed to the cost of long-term care for a chronic condition. In doing so, they set the stage for higher costs, even denial of coverage, for those who fail to comply with such healthy pursuits (Miller 2009, pers. comm.). Julianne Cheek (2008: 981), borrowing from Yoder, notes that in the era of biomedicalization, 'people are blamed for both their acts and their omissions – what they do wrong and what they fail to do right'. Health as a responsibility, rather than a right, repositions subjects as at fault if they are deemed unhealthy, particularly if they had the information about how to achieve health. (As if it were that formulaic.)

Guthman and DuPuis (2006: 444) argue that public-health interventions that work on the population level aim to divide and conquer – to 'prevent, contain, or eliminate the abnormal'. Those remaining 'healthy' are then recognized as superior to their problematic counterparts.

Neoliberal governmentality produces contradictory impulses such that the neoliberal subject is emotionally compelled to participate in society as both out-of-control consumer and self-controlled subject. The perfect subject-citizen is able to achieve both eating and thinness, even if having it both ways entails eating nonfoods of questionable health impact or throwing up the food one does eat. Those who can achieve thinness amidst this plenty are imbued with the rationality and self-discipline that those who are fat must logically lack; they then become the deserving in a political economy all too geared toward legitimizing such distinctions.

(Guthman and DuPuis 2006: 444)

In the context of excess that characterizes the era and sites of neoliberal governance, we revere moderation – we celebrate those who want *less*. However, as Guthman and DuPuis (2006) point out, wanting less alone is no longer the mark of salvation that it was for the Puritans.[2] Instead, the neoliberal citizen is charged with wanting less but at the same time spending more (Guthman and DuPuis 2006: 445).

State interventions in obesity

I want to return for a moment to the news story and accompanying advertisement that I described at the opening of this chapter. Part of what is happening there seems to be just this very spectacle of censure and contradiction. We are invited to empathize with neither the fat teenager nor the desperate mother on the lam; instead, with phrases like 'medical neglect' and 'fugitive' looming large, we immediately recognize these people (who are, not coincidentally, working-class people of colour – perhaps invoking cultural memories of the mythic welfare queen and the dangerous black male youth) as Other. We can set ourselves up, then, in contrast: as healthy, appropriate, moderate consumers. The Wendy's ad speaks to us, reminds us of our distinction from the undifferentiated masses whose inability to manage their own risks and control their own bodies means that sometimes the state has to step in. The state has 'empowered' the mother to help her son lose weight, in a move reminiscent of McNaughton's observation of 'new opportunities for surveillance, regulation and disciplining of "threatening" (fat) maternal bodies' (this volume; see also Ristovski-Slijepcevic, this volume). If she can't or won't, the will to empower and to manage risk trumps familial bonding.

Petersen (2003: 193) argues that 'the notion of empowerment and the techniques of risk have come to play a crucial role as techniques and technologies of governance, in shaping the conduct of individuals in ways which make them more self-governing'. It is in this light that we must examine public-health interventions like those described earlier in this chapter that, using various forms of surveillance, are designed to empower the individual (which nearly always translates to making that individual lose weight). The Alexander Draper case is not purely a public-health intervention; it is about a lot of other things, including child welfare and parental rights and responsibilities – but you had better believe that it sounds an ominous note about the importance of heeding the seemingly benign (or, more generously, benevolent) public-health information circulated through our culture in myriad forms. The Draper case, and others like it, shows us the unpleasant consequences of failure to submit to norms of biomedical self-governance.

But if Draper is the endpoint, there is a good deal of backing up we must do to consider the 'chances' the state gives its citizens to make the 'good choices' about their bodies that would, presumably, prevent or cure obesity. Legislation like Mississippi's House Bill 282, which proposed refusing to serve food to fat people in restaurants, was arguably an object lesson rather than an earnest attempt at law-making (Tate 2008). One of the legislators involved stated that the bill was serious, but admitted that it may have been more aimed at drawing attention to the obesity epidemic 'in the hopes that one or two people will sit up and take notice to make the necessary lifestyle changes to lead a healthy life' (Tate 2008: n.p.).

Likewise, as I mentioned earlier, there have been many efforts at the state level to pass BMI bills that would require, variously, in-school weigh-ins, physical fitness tests and nutrition education. Many of these school-based public-health campaigns are designed to alleviate risk. According to O'Bryne and Holmes (2007: 99):

> Risk becomes an excellent yardstick by which citizens can be ranked as good or bad. Individuals who engage in activities that may put them or others at risk are bad citizens who must be made aware of their status through health-related mass-media campaigns. Furthermore, by the encouragement of annual health examinations, individuals are persuaded to submit their bodies and their practices to the gaze of an expert who will perform a more individualized assessment, thereby providing a more exact ranking of the individual as in good or bad health.

Such laws that require individualized assessments of children by experts exist in six US states, while in others they did not quite make it through the legislative process but spent considerable time on the docket. Those that do exist usually involve the creation of health and wellness councils populated by all members of the school community (teachers, students, parents, food service staff, health professionals and so on); these councils serve in an advisory capacity to create and monitor nutrition and physical activity rules and practices. The bills usually mandate numerous forms of nutrition and physical education that emphasize the importance of maintaining a healthy weight and teach how to accomplish that via eating and exercise. Through these efforts, the state (via its institutional apparatus, the public school) responsibilizes the citizenry, providing information and opportunity that any rational, in-control actor would of course take to protect his or her own health.

The consequences of a negative 'BMI Report Card' or 'Fitnessgram' are not as widely publicized. One Philadelphia hospital website takes an upbeat approach, advising parents how to deal with a child whose BMI Report Card shows that they are overweight or obese: call the school nurse to find out what the school is doing to help; call the child's doctor who might advise you to alter your family's TV viewing, eating and exercise patterns; and involve the whole family:

> Don't single out this child as having an individual problem, because the entire family's leisure time and eating habits could probably be improved. That approach also avoids psychological harm to your child. You don't want your child to feel mortified. You also don't want to raise your child's odds of developing an eating disorder.
> (Hahnemann University Hospital 2008: n.p.)

In Arkansas, where they considered repealing their BMI bill, Governor Mike Beebe claimed that school weigh-ins and report cards had many negative, unintended consequences and damaged some children's self-esteem. Unlike his predecessor, the formerly fat anti-obesity presidential campaigner Mike Huckabee, Beebe favours an easy parental opt-out and wanted to reduce the frequency of weight-testing (Newsmax 2007: n.p.). It seems surprising that in a child-centred era where self-esteem is paramount and considered to be essential to well-rounded selfhood, the best we can come up with in terms of public-health interventions has a great capacity to shame young people (Scheier 2004) – surely not the best cornerstone of a healthy population (yet with plenty of precedent in parallel tobacco-control efforts; see McCullough, this volume; West 2007; Bell *et al.* 2009).

Another prong of many anti-obesity public-health interventions is school-lunch reform. While there are many good reasons one might want to change the food and foodways of schools (catsup is not a vegetable, industrial food has profoundly negative environmental and economic effects, cults of branded consumerism, etc.), school-lunch reformers tend to zero in on only one: obesity (see Food Museum 2005 for but one example). Reform is not just about removing junk food from cafeterias, but about inculcating a sense of 'ownership' of food in children – sometimes by launching participatory gardening and cooking programmes, by changing the dining atmosphere, and by exciting curricular revisions that give kids taste-buds-on experience with new foods. This is what Share and Strain (2008: 242) might call 'young people engage[ing] with technologies of power through institutionalised democratic forms of participation and active engagement with school governance', a wonderful alternative to top-down direction by the state. These all seem like great ideas in and of themselves – yay for cooking! yay for gardening! yay for tasting fresh tomatoes in class! – but they make me wary when they are enlisted simply to combat obesity. It is as if fatness is such a terrifying spectre in the cultural imaginary that only its threat could motivate us to change a deeply flawed food system. But what happens when we make these changes, and some people remain fat, as some people have been fat since the dawn of time?

Even though revisionist school-lunch programmes have been invented in part to combat a growing 'obesity epidemic' among children and thus to improve their health, there is no real proof that better food at school has such effects (Belkin 2006). 'We don't have these children 24 hours a day,' says researcher Benjamin Caballero. 'They go home, they go out with friends, they are off all summer and everything about the world – fast food, video games, television ads, everything – conspires to undo even the best things that happen in schools' (Belkin 2006: n.p.). This comment suggests the extent to which the state/public-health folks *would* like to have the children all the time – extending their reach and power when parents and friends and culture in general cannot be counted on to keep them in line. Belkin's article also mentions a school in Florida that exiles children who eat junk food to have lunch outdoors (which sounds lovely until one remembers that Kissimmee is ungodly hot, and that it still rains quite a lot in the Sunshine State) because of a ban on junk food in the cafeteria. Surely, such social isolation brings few promises of health.

Alternatives to neoliberal governmentality and the obesogenic environment account

Much scholarship that is wise or critical about governmentality points out the problem with seeing the individual healthcare consumer as rational and unbound by larger social structure (see Petersen 2003; Williams 2003; Broom 2008). A chorus of voices has responded critically to the way in which neoliberal governmentality shifts responsibility for the 'problem' of obesity onto the individual, who is tasked with the making of 'good choices'. But the upshot of such a critique, when applied to the 'problem of obesity', is sometimes – often – a strenuously renewed effort on remediating the obesogenic environments which allegedly contribute to obesity (which is collapsed into ill-health, as noted earlier) (see Critser 2003; Yancey *et al.* 2006; Berlant 2007; Elliott 2007; Share and Strain 2008).

This is not a route I want to take. Such scholars and public-health advocates prefer to focus on changing the 'obesogenic environment' that makes 'good choices' impossible for marginalized segments of the population. They note that 'good choices' edicts aimed broadly may have the effect of widening health disparities, as the inevitable failure of some people (the poor, the elderly, disabled people, people of colour, etc.) who lack recourse to structural supports for those 'good choices' will itself, because of our cultural expectations about personal accountability, elicit further stigmatization and punishment by those who *do* capably control their bodies.

In contrast, I aim to, first, reconfigure and de-pathologize fatness away from its present formulation of medicalized 'obesity epidemic'; second, to unhinge fatness from its seemingly (and incorrectly) necessary relationship with ill-health; and third, to problematize our moral imperative for health.

What does one think of when one thinks of an epidemic? Usually, it is the potential for contagion (Elliott 2007). Although a recent medical study has suggested just that – that contact with fat people lessens inhibitions about becoming fat (Christakis and Fowler 2007) – this takes 'contagion' to have a different meaning than the old germ theory usage. Medical researchers Christakis and Fowler substitute 'contagion' for what they really mean ('social influence') because it extends the language and the metaphor of the 'obesity epidemic'. The very language of 'epidemic' when applied to the phenomenon of fatness invites a response that is self-protective (for those of average weight) and that requires the monitoring of (and distancing from) fat others. This does not make a whole lot of sense to me as a way to make people healthier. Instead, it seems to me that the effect on fat people of pathologizing fatness is primarily a heightened sense of shame (Christian 2007), an aversion to seeking medical care when it is really necessary (Maiman *et al.* 1979; Culbertson and Smollen 1999), and the cultivation of unhealthy relationships to food including binge eating, extreme dieting and rampant weight cycling (Berg 1993; Germov and Williams 1996) that have been shown to have more deleterious health effects than a stable but high weight.

Although it is a challenging act of imagination in an environment supersaturated with 'obesity epidemic' rhetoric, I would like us to think of fatness as a form of human diversity. Why does fat have to be unhealthy? If one reconceptualizes fatness as a typical human variation in body size and shape, rather than pathologizing it, the causal links to ill-health and even death that have been scaled back or undermined (Flegal *et al.* 2005) seem tenuous at best.[3] If one insists on punishing people who do not religiously perform self-restraint by tarring them with the label 'unhealthy' before one has even investigated their habits of eating and movement and their vitals, the 'obesity epidemic' is a convenient vehicle for castigation. But for those with a *genuine* interest in health – rather than a desire to use concerns about health as a smokescreen for moral judgements and social condemnation – there is much to be gained by thinking about fat bodies more neutrally, rather than presuming a transparency that says the body size and shape tells us everything we need to know about a person's health. Plenty of us know thin or average-weight people with terrible eating habits who never exercise – yet they are not subject to the same conclusions about their health or their moral worthiness, because they do not wear what we take to be the evidence of excessive consumption on their bodies (LeBesco 2004). Some fat people are healthy, and some fat people are not. If we really want good health for all, we must stop assuming otherwise.

Nearly thirty years ago, Robert Crawford (1980) coined the term 'healthism' – a political ideology that elevates healthy lifestyle to a high moral calling – to describe the phenomenon we are now seeing very much at work in public responses to what critics now describe as our slight collective weight gain (Campos 2004), rather than some sign of the apocalypse. Crawford's work was extended by Petr Skrabanek (1994), who argues that healthism has underpinned racism and eugenic campaigns that separate the 'healthy' (which equates to moral and pure) from the 'unhealthy' (the foreign or impure). While Skrabanek worried that the state's embrace of 'lifestylism' effectively gave the state unlimited coercive/prescriptive power around issues of health, Rose (1999), following Foucault (1991), instead emphasized the hegemonic character of healthism: the state does not need to *make* people be healthy, as the citizens of course *want* to be healthy, partly as the condition of living in a society that profoundly marginalizes those who 'opt out' of health.

This discussion has important implications for thinking about the lived experience of fatness. With few exceptions, the state does not compel people to lose weight by force. Rather, our capitalist culture industries make it rather unappealing to be fat, so much so that most fat people internalize this stigma and admit to a sincere desire to be thinner. We pay lip service to the idea that 'beauty is in the eye of the beholder', and seem to realize that condemning fat people because we do not like how they look is just plain rude. (Not to mention immoral: 'Judge not lest ye be judged' says the gospel according to Matthew.) We need a more compelling argument. And voilà, exhorting them to change because 'fat is just so unhealthy!' puts us on safe moral ground. We're not being mean – we're helping, striving for a better society of well and vigorous individuals by giving people information about their health risks and possibilities for prevention and treatment. We're giving them choices about how to proceed! We're looking out for our brothers and sisters!

The problem is that the very policing of fatness on health grounds endangers the well-being of fat people. Petersen (2003: 195) observes that:

> There has been little discussion about the individual's right *not* to know and the right *not* to choose, since this would run counter to the imperative to be an active decision-maker and would throw into question the legitimacy of the compulsory structures which compel an agent to behave in particular ways. Those who seek to operate outside predetermined lines of action risk being labelled irresponsible or as troublemakers and suffering financial penalty of some kind or being denied access to services or advice. In other words, the range of possible ethical actions is always circumscribed (although not determined) by the imperatives of rule.

Fat people, whether their fatness is an agentic 'no' to biopower or a more ambivalent, less baldly volitional experience of embodied resistance, clearly operate outside the predetermined lines of action that Petersen describes. He suggests a way forward, outside the lines of biomedical governmentality, in advancing an individual's right *not* to know and *not* to choose in a saturated information environment that enables 'good choices' and punishes bad ones. Decentring health as the be-all, end-all of human subjectivity is the task ahead of us. We need to think critically about what Markula (2008: n.p.) describes as 'the largely economic premise for the panic of the obesity epidemic' rather than swallowing whole meaningless, manipulable statistics from questionably reliable and arguably invalid epidemiological research (Clough 2004). It seems to me that we need to look more closely at paths to well-being that abstain from the kind of carrot and stick model that beats down those it pre-emptively deems unhealthy.[4] It is this model that is making me, and many, many others, sick.

Notes

1 Responsibilization is 'the social process that imposes specific responsibilities on some category of social agents' (Rous and Hunt 2004: 826).
2 Bunton (this volume) effectively complicates our understandings of the Puritan stance towards pleasure.
3 Even after the Centers for Disease Control significantly scaled back its estimate of the impact of overweight and obesity on mortality rates in 2005, CDC Director Julie Gerberding declined to use the new figure in CDC public-awareness campaigns (*The Medical News* 2005). This evidences a vehement commitment to obesity epidemic rhetoric, 'facts' be damned.
4 One such possible path is the Health at Every Size (HAES) movement (see LeBesco 2010). Whereas governmentality scholars have been criticized for paying inadequate attention to resistance to biomedical regimes (Petersen 2003), a focus on HAES and similar initiatives allows us to 'recognise the ways in which subjects, individually and collectively, tactically deploy the practices and products imposed on them to achieve particular ends' (Petersen 2003: 198). But whereas Petersen champions such resistance, some public-health scholars (e.g. Broom 2008) worry that such oppositionality might exacerbate health conditions in a cut-off-one's-nose-to-spite-one's-face kind of manoeuvre. In contrast, I believe that we have to leave room for the possibility that such oppositionality is part of what keeps people sane and healthy in a pathologizing environment.

References

Bacchi, C. and Beasley, C. (2002) 'Citizen bodies: Is embodied citizenship a contradiction in terms?', *Critical Social Policy*, 22(2): 324–352.
Belkin, L. (2006) 'The school lunch test', *New York Times Magazine*. Online, available at: www.nytimes.com/2006/08/20/magazine/20lunches.html?pagewanted =1& r=1 (accessed 28 June 2009).
Bell, K., McNaughton, D. and Salmon, A. (2009) 'Medicine, morality and mothering: Public health discourses on foetal alcohol exposure, smoking around children and childhood overnutrition', *Critical Public Health*, 19(2): 155–170.
Berg, F. (1993) *The Health Risks of Obesity* (Healthy Living Institute), Hettinger: Decker Periodicals.

Berlant, L. (2007) 'Slow death', *Critical Inquiry*, 33: 754–780.

Broom, D. (2008) 'Hazardous good intentions? Unintended consequences of the project of prevention', *Health Sociology Review*, 17(2): 129–140.

Campos, P. (2004) *The Obesity Myth*, New York: Gotham.

Campos, P., Saguy, A., Ernsberger, P., Oliver, E. and Gaesser, G. (2006) 'The epidemiology of overweight and obesity: Public health crisis or moral panic?', *International Journal of Epidemiology*, 35: 55–60.

Cheek, J. (2008) 'Healthism: A new conservatism?', *Qualitative Health Research*, 18(7): 974–982.

Christakis, N.A. and Fowler, J.H. (2007) 'The spread of obesity in a large social network over 32 years', *The New England Journal of Medicine*, 357(4): 370–379.

Christian, N. (2007) 'Shame game "losing" war on obesity', *Scotland on Sunday*. Online, available at: http://scotlandonsunday.scotsman.com/obesity/Shame-game-losing-war-on.3309001.jp (accessed 30 June 2009).

Clough, P.T. (2004) 'Technoscience, global politics, and cultural criticism', *Social Text*, 22(3): 1–23.

Coveney, J. (2008) 'The government of girth', *Health Sociology Review*, 17(2): 199–214.

Crawford, R. (1980) 'Healthism and the medicalization of everyday life', *International Journal of Health Services*, 10(3): 365–388.

Critser, G. (2003) *Fat Land: How Americans Became the Fattest People in the World*, Boston: Houghton Mifflin.

Culbertson, M. and Smolen, M. (1999) 'Attitudes toward personalities and lifestyles of obese adults', *Journal of Nursing Education*, 38(2): 84.

Dean, M. (1999) *Governmentality: Power and Rule in Modern Society*, Thousand Oaks: Sage.

Elliott, C.D. (2007) 'Big persons, small voices: On governance, obesity, and the narrative of the failed citizen', *Journal of Canadian Studies*, 41(3): 134–149.

Flegal, K.M., Graubard, B.I., Williamson, D.F. and Gail, M.H. (2005) 'Excess deaths associated with underweight, overweight, and obesity', *Journal of the American Medical Association*, 293(15): 1861–1867.

Food Museum (2005) 'School lunch reform', *The FOOD Museum Online*. Online, available at: www.foodmuseum.com/issuesschoollunch.html (accessed 30 June 2009).

Foucault, M. (1975) *Discipline and Punish*, New York: Random House.

Foucault, M. (1991) 'The ethic of care for the self as a practice of freedom: An interview with Michel Foucault on January 20, 1984', in J. Bernauer and D. Rasmussen (eds) *The Final Foucault*, Cambridge, MA: MIT Press, pp. 1–20.

Fox Carolina (2009) 'Missing 555-pound teen found in Maryland: Mother faces charge in SC', *FoxCarolina.com*. Online, available at: www.foxcarolina.com/news/19528330/detail.html (accessed 28 June 2009).

Gard, M. and Wright, J. (2005) *The Obesity Epidemic: Science, Morality and Ideology*, New York: Routledge.

Georgia General Assembly (2008) 'Senate bill 506, SHAPE Act', *Georgia General Assembly*. Online, available at: www.legis.state.ga.us/legis/2007_08/sum/sb506.htm (accessed 28 June 2009).

Germov, J. and Williams, L. (1996) 'The epidemic of dieting women: The need for a sociological approach to food and nutrition', *Appetite*, 27: 97–108.

Guthman, J. and DuPuis, M. (2006) 'Embodying neoliberalism: Economy, culture, and the politics of fat', *Environment and Planning D: Society and Space*, 24: 427–448.

Hahnemann University Hospital (2008) 'Report cards "grade" kids' weight', *Hahnemann University Hospital*. Online, available at: http://hahnemannhospital. staywellsolutionsonline.com/RelatedItems/1,4188 (accessed 29 June 2009).

Jutel, A. (2005) 'Weighing health: The moral burden of obesity', *Social Semiotics*, 15(2): 113–125.

LeBesco, K. (2004) *Revolting Bodies? The Struggle to Redefine Fat Identity*, Amherst: University of Massachusetts Press.

LeBesco, K. (2010) 'Fat panic and the invisible morality', in J. Metzl and A. Kirkland (eds) *Against Health: A Manifesto*, New York: New York University Press, pp. 72–82.

Levenstein, H. (2003) *Paradox of Plenty: A Social History of Eating in Modern America, Revised Edition*, Berkeley: University of California Press.

Maiman, L., Wang, V., Beckler, M., Finlay, J. and Simonson, M. (1979) 'Attitudes toward obesity and the obese among professionals', *Journal of the American Dietetic Association*, 74: 331–336.

Markula, P. (2008) 'Governing obese bodies in a control society', *Junctures: The Journal for Thematic Dialogue*, 11: 53–66.

The Medical News (2005) 'Overweight not as bad as once thought', *The Medical News*. Online, available at: www.news-medical.net/news/2005/04/20/9393.aspx (accessed 29 June 2009).

Miller, C. (2009) Personal communication with author, 29 June.

Mississippi Legislature (2008) 'House bill 282, 2008', *Mississippi Legislature, Regular Session*. Online, available at: http://billstatus.ls.state.ms.us/2008/pdf/ history/HB/HB0282.xml (accessed 28 June 2009).

Murray, S. (2005) '(Un/be)coming out? Rethinking fat politics', *Social Semiotics*, 15(2): 153–163.

New York City Department of Education (2006) 'NYC Department of Education wellness policies on physical activity and nutrition', *Healthy Lunches.org*. Online, available at: www.healthylunches.org/docs/NewYorkCityWellnessPolicy200607_English.pdf (accessed 28 June 2009).

Newsmax (2007) 'Arkansas may ditch obesity report cards for kids', *Newsmax.com*. Online, available at: http://archive.newsmax.com/archives/articles/2007/2/6/121254. shtml (accessed 30 June 2009).

O'Byrne, P. and Holmes, D. (2007) 'The micro-fascism of Plato's good citizen: Producing (dis)order through the construction of risk', *Nursing Philosophy*, 8: 92–101.

Petersen, A. (2003) 'Governmentality, critical scholarship, and the medical humanities', *Journal of Medical Humanities*, 24(3/4): 187–201.

Rose, N. (1999) *Powers of Freedom: Reframing Political Thought*, Cambridge: Cambridge University Press.

Rous, R. and Hunt, A. (2004) 'Governing peanuts: The regulation of the social bodies of children and the risks of food allergies', *Social Science and Medicine*, 58: 825–836.

Saguy, A.C. and Riley, K.W. (2005) 'Weighing both sides: Morality, mortality, and framing contests over obesity', *Journal of Health Politics, Policy and Law*, 30(5): 869–921.

Scheier, L.M. (2004) 'Potential problems with school health report cards', *Journal of the American Dietetic Association*, 104(4): 525–527.

Share, M. and Strain, M. (2008) 'Making schools and young people responsible: A critical analysis of Ireland's obesity strategy', *Health and Social Care in the Community*, 16(3): 234–243.

Skrabanek, P. (1994) *The Death of Humane Medicine and the Rise of Coercive Healthism*, Edmunds: Social Affairs Unit.

Tate, A. (2008) 'Obesity and Mississippi's House of Representatives Bill 282', *Associated Content, Health and Wellness*. Online, available at: www.associated-content.com/article/583883/obesity_and_mississippis_house_of_representatives.html?cat=5 (accessed 30 June 2009).

West, R. (2007) 'What lessons can be learned from tobacco control for combating the growing prevalence of obesity', *Obesity Reviews*, 8(1): 145–150.

Whyte, S.R. (2009) 'Health identities and subjectivities: The ethnographic challenge', *Medical Anthropology Quarterly*, 23(1): 6–15.

Williams, G.H. (2003) 'The determinants of health: Structure, context and agency', *Sociology of Health and Illness*, 25(3): 131–154.

Yancey, A.K., Leslie, J. and Abel, E.K. (2006) 'Obesity at the crossroads: Feminist and public health perspectives', *Signs*, 31(2): 425–443.

3 Addiction and personal responsibility as solutions to the contradictions of neoliberal consumerism[1]

Robin Room

Alcohol as a consumer good

Present-day industrial and post-industrial societies have built their economies around consumption. Economists sometimes divide consumer goods into those characterized by 'inventory adjustment' and those that are 'habit forming' (Houtthakker and Taylor 1970). Purchasing a refrigerator or an axe today predicts I will not purchase it tomorrow. So demand for such goods eventually reaches a limit in a given population, with further purchases being primarily replacements – adjustments of the inventory. On the other hand, purchase of a habit-forming good today predicts I will purchase it tomorrow. Demand for inventory-adjustment goods is thus inherently limited in a way that demand for habit-forming goods is not.

As a quintessential habit-forming commodity, alcohol, along with other psychoactive substances, is thus ideal for building and sustaining markets. Increasingly large-scale beer and spirits production featured in the early stages of European industrialization (e.g. Bennett 1999; Caldwell 1996). In the centuries of European colonial expansion, alcoholic beverages, along with other psychoactive substances, became part of the 'glue of empires' (Courtwright 2001): a favoured trade good, since it created its own demand; and often an instrument for exploitation of labour (Crush and Ambler 1992; Room *et al.* 2002: 22–27). In home markets, too, the 'gin epidemic' in England and equivalent episodes in other European countries pushed consumption to very high levels.

The demand for sober attention and the rise and fall of temperance

On the other hand, the Industrial Revolution created, and modern life has increased, the demand for consciousness, attention and conscientiousness. Historical analyses have described the gradual separation between work and leisure as part of the Industrial Revolution (Gusfield 1991), with the accompanying demand for attention and frequently for meticulousness at work. Modern life has added other circumstances in which exacting attention is demanded. While driving a car is the most obvious such circumstance, there are also others. Modern societies, for instance, expect attention and conscientiousness of parents in charge of small children to a degree that would surprise eighteenth-century observers.

Drinking alcohol is a clear threat to these demands. Even a few drinks threatens attention and impairs coordination and judgement. Habitual drinking tends to impair performance of major social roles, particularly in family and work life. Two centuries ago, however, social customs overrode any such consideration. Drinking was intimately entwined in the working day among skilled tradesmen in the early nineteenth century (Adler 1991). Hogarth's famous print 'Gin Lane' illustrates the extent to which the heavy drinking of the time obstructed parental responsibilities.

The adverse effects of drinking on work and home life were major considerations in the delayed societal response to the heavy drinking of the eighteenth and early nineteenth centuries, which took the form of the temperance movements of the nineteenth and early twentieth centuries. Many of these temperance movements first gained strength primarily as self-help movements among skilled workers (e.g. Harrison 1971), but nineteenth-century industrialists enthusiastically joined the cause, seeking a sober workforce (Rosenzweig 1983; Rumbarger 1989). Perhaps the most lasting achievement of the temperance movement in English-speaking countries was largely to remove alcohol from the workplace.

The international temperance movement reached its zenith during and in the years immediately after the First World War, attaining full prohibition of alcohol in the US, Canada, Finland, Russia, and briefly in Norway and Iceland. Then its strength began to wane. What had seemed a progressive cause to university students in 1910 had become for the students of the 1930s something to rebel against as old-fashioned (Room 1984b). In the fiscal crisis of the Depression, many industrialists also turned against Prohibition, putting a greater priority on the potential contribution of alcohol sales to the economy and of alcohol taxes to government revenue than on sobriety in the workforce (Levine 1985).

The temperance era left behind in English-speaking and some other countries strong structures of state control over the alcohol market, in many places initially including personalized controls over purchasing and consumption. These structures, which today would be called 'harm-reduction' measures, were often adopted in the teeth of temperance movement opposition, but in response to its pressure (Room 2004a). Until 1955, sale of spirits by the bottle was limited in Sweden to purchase of a personalized ration (Mäkelä et al. 2002). In several Canadian provinces, there were limits on how much could be purchased at a time, and an 'interdict list' of those forbidden to purchase; in Ontario until the 1960s, purchasers left a signed record of their purchases (Room et al. 2006). In a wider spread of places, the market was subject to general limits on availability which did not single out the individual purchaser or drinker, including limited hours of sale and limits on the number of sales outlets (Babor *et al.* 2010, chapter 9).

The retreat from alcohol control and its rationales

In the many places in which strong alcohol control systems were set up between 1915 and 1935, the past sixty years have seen a lengthy retreat, with specific commercial interests and consumer-sovereignty and free-market ideologies pushing always towards a more open market (Room 2010). For many years, the primary argument justifying this was in terms, on the one hand, of consumer convenience, and on the other, of a distinction between the 'alcoholic' and the social drinker. The alcoholic, it was argued, was a sick person subject to a 'predisposing X factor' (Jellinek 1952), whether due to genes or upbringing. As a sick person, the alcoholic deserved treatment (Room 1983). But that was no reason for the rest of us 'normal drinkers' to be subject to restrictive controls. The new 'alcoholism movement', devoted to providing treatment for the alcoholic and to research on alcoholism, was therefore largely welcomed and supported by the alcoholic-beverage industry (Rubin 1979). The alcoholism movement, in turn, gladly lent its expertise to enquiries and legislative hearings which concluded that the system of alcohol controls should be partly abandoned (e.g. Bracken 1955). The Alcoholism Research Foundation of Ontario, now part of the Centre for Addiction and Mental Health, was set up in 1949 to provide treatment for alcoholics effectively as a quid pro quo for the introduction of liquor-by-the-drink (alcohol in bars and restaurants; Archibald 1990). Likewise, 'Saskatchewan and Manitoba set up Alcoholism Commissions to build a provincial [alcoholism] treatment system in direct connection with legalizing cocktail bars, cabarets and liquor licenses for restaurants' (Room *et al.* 2006: 22). An analysis looking back in 1981 concluded that 'the expansion of the [alcoholism] treatment system may be seen as a kind of cultural alibi' for the relaxation of controls on the alcohol market (Mäkelä *et al.* 1981: 65).

By the 1980s, the alcoholism paradigm as an explanation of the whole range of alcohol problems was losing some steam, in the face of a competing 'new public health model' which recognized the diversity of alcohol-related problems and defended the utility of alcohol controls (Room 1984a; Sutton 1998). In recent years, there has also been some shifting in the public discourse about alcohol problems away from alcoholism to intoxication. Problems of intoxication – drink-driving casualties, fighting on the streets, unwanted sex – presently dominate daily media coverage of alcohol issues in the UK and Australia (e.g. Wilkinson 2008). At the intellectual level, the emphasis of the new public-health model on the overall population level of consumption has been attacked in favour of an emphasis on intoxication events as the source of most alcohol problems (e.g. Stockwell *et al.* 1997).

The shift to an emphasis on drinking-in-the-event rather than chronic drinking-as-a-condition was to some extent foreshadowed by concerns about drink-driving, which reached a first peak in the 1960s. In that era, a stricter regime on drink-driving was sometimes the quid pro quo for relaxation of alcohol controls. Thus a statutory 0.05 per cent blood alcohol limit for driving was recommended in the same 1965 commission report in the Australian state of Victoria that called for abandoning the six o'clock limit on closing time for pubs (Boorman 1999). Both proposals became law. More recently, it is concerns about intoxicated street behaviour that have brought political initiatives to deter and punish individual offenders through such mechanisms as Anti-Social Behaviour Orders (ASBOs) in the UK and 'banning orders' in Victoria (Consumer Affairs 2007; Room 2004c).

The contradictions of alcohol in the consumer society, and their resolutions

As Bunton (this volume) notes in other terms, there is thus a contradiction built into the ideology of consumer sovereignty as applied to alcohol in modern societies. As a habit-forming psychoactive substance, alcohol tends to build and sustain its own demand. However, consumption of more than a limited amount disables the user for the consciousness, attention and conscientiousness demanded of major roles – as a worker, as a parent, as a driver, and for that matter as a person using public space.

One resolution of this contradiction is to forbid use of the psychoactive substance. Such a prohibition is the solution of present-day societies for such substances as cocaine, heroin and cannabis. A second resolution, applied for many other psychoactive substances used, is regulation by a prescription regime which strongly limits availability, putting doctors in charge of an individualized rationing scheme. For alcohol, however, each of these solutions have been out of favour in Western societies for eighty years.

A third resolution, a weaker form of the second, is a strong control system that seeks to hold down consumption levels and tries in many ways to reduce harm from the substance use. This was the solution adopted for alcohol at the repeal of prohibition in societies where there had been a period of prohibition, and in some other societies also (Room 2004a).

The fourth resolution is to treat the substance as an ordinary commodity, subject to the rules on marketing and availability for commodities in general.[2] It is inherent in this resolution that all responsibility for resolving the contradiction is placed on the individual drinker. When alcohol problems were primarily conceptualized in terms of alcoholism, the responsibility was to avoid developing a habit of regular heavy drinking, i.e. to avoid becoming alcohol-dependent or alcoholic. As attention has increasingly turned to alcohol-in-the-event, the responsibility is increasingly conceptualized in terms of avoiding intoxication. An early exponent of this, Morris Chafetz, later the first director of the US National Institute on Alcohol Abuse and Alcoholism, specified in 1967 that anyone who 'has been intoxicated four times in a year' should be considered a problem drinker (Chafetz 1967). Similarly, arguments from alcohol industry sources touting the advantages of drinking have been careful to specify that it is *moderate* drinking, and not intoxication, that they favour: 'Citizens for Moderation [represents] the interests of [those] who consume responsibly and in good health' (Citizens for Moderation 1989).

A special case of placing the responsibility on the individual drinker is the injunction on pregnant women to avoid drinking, regardless of how alcoholized may be the social context in which they find themselves. Bell *et al.* (2009) have noted the moralization of drinking in pregnancy as a threat to the health of the infant, and Salmon (this volume) discusses the specific application of this frame with respect to Aboriginal Canadians. France requires a warning label or a logo of a slash over a pregnant woman holding a glass on alcoholic-beverage containers, and the world's second-largest distiller has moved to extend such warning labels to the whole European Union (Mercer 2006). From the beverage industry's perspective, pregnant women are a small market; giving way in this area may distract from any measures that might have broader impact.

The strait path of moderate drinking: the new pilgrim's progress

Intoxication has remained morally reprehensible or at least questionable in most mainstream public discourse throughout the modern period. Those on the 'wetter' side of debates about drinking practices and policies have been at pains to differentiate controlled or moderate drinking from intoxication, and to assign opposite moral valences to them – negative for intoxication, but positive for controlled or moderate drinking. The moralization of controlled or moderate drinking thus derives in the first place from the contrast with intoxication and intoxicated bad behaviour.

But arguments for controlled or moderate drinking often seem to invest it with further moral significance. In the framing of the cognitive behavioural psychologists who have argued for 'controlled drinking' as a goal for those in treatment for problematic drinking, moderation in drinking becomes a positive good in itself, a moral and personal achievement on the part of the drinker. Thus Marlatt (1985: 329, 332) argues for moderation as 'the key to lifestyle balance', as well as on the utilitarian ground that it 'enhances pleasure at the least cost to the individual'. For Marlatt (1985: 333, 334), 'moderation represents a balance point or border area between the extremes of absolute restraint or control and loss of control (addiction).... Moderation and a flexible attitude contrasts sharply with excessive constraint and *overcontrol*.'

Such arguments assert or imply a moral superiority of moderate or controlled drinking over abstention from drinking as well as over intoxication. The superiority is demonstrated by the drinker's successful self-control in the course of each drinking occasion. 'From a moderation perspective, control implies *choice*.... Moderation implies learning to "take it or leave it" whereas control (and overcontrol) in the traditional sense implies only the option to leave (abstain)' (Marlatt 1985: 335). As a corollary of this line of thinking, moderate drinking should be engaged in with some regularity to demonstrate its controlled nature. Thus the normative ideal of moderate or controlled drinking takes on a frequency as well as a quantity dimension. As Duckert (1989: 40) notes, 'the most common demand for "controlled drinking" is that it should take place in the form of some high-frequency low-dosage consumption'; Stockwell's (1986) 'criteria for controlled drinking', for instance, include drinking at least once a week.

Behind the arguments for moderate or controlled drinking can be discerned the outlines of a new version of an old worldview – of the passage through daily life as a series of tests and trials of character – a view deep-set in Protestant-influenced cultures through such religious antecedents as Bunyan's *Pilgrim's Progress*. In this modern and secularized version of the pilgrim's progress, it is drinking behaviour that becomes a daily test of character. By drinking moderately or in a controlled fashion, the modern pilgrim exercises and demonstrates his or her self-control and rationality in a new trial every day.

> A particularly heavy burden that society places on the individual is the demand for self-control. By *self-control* we mean the exercise of a controlling response or strategy ... [on] behavior that is either very firmly established as a long time habit or momentarily attractive, ... [behavior that is] usually easy to execute but disadvantageous in the long run.... Moderation is prescribed by society for many [such] behaviors. Diverse interest groups, however, flourish in our societies and some thrive on producing or exalting behaviors and products that tempt the flesh, the mind, and the palate.... [While] social rules and etiquette guide proper timing, frequency, and quantity of alcohol consumption, ... nevertheless each person is ultimately held responsible for monitoring their judicious use of alcohol, and expected to control drinking within defined ranges and on specified occasions.
>
> (Kanfer 1986: 30–31)

The underlying worldview of controlled or moderate drinking as an ideology and programme of ostensive self-control ties together three separate arguments. One of these is a valuation of moderate drinking over abstention. By abstaining, one is opting out of the test altogether, choosing the soft option rather than a more exacting test of one's self-control. The second aspect is the negative valence on intoxication. This aspect is so taken for granted that it is often not explicitly discussed. The third aspect is an aversion to state intervention in the alcohol market. Graham (1996: xvii), for instance, argues against 'restricting the general availability of alcohol' on two grounds: 'the futility of trying to keep ... addicts away from the substance they crave', and 'being grossly unfair to those who drink moderately'. From the perspective of valorizing controlled/moderate drinking as a unifying worldview, if the state facilitates controlled or moderate drinking by controlling the conditions of sale of alcohol, it is undercutting the trial and display of good moral character involved in drinking.

With respect to the alcohol market, the state is thus viewed as a pitiful helpless giant: even if it can accomplish anything in this area, it will be counterproductive, by diminishing the role for personal responsibility and demonstrations of self-control. The proper role of the state, in this view, is limited to punishing those who have failed the moral test of responsible drinking. Thus, vigorous state action is called for in 'holding people responsible for their drug use and other behavior'; 'jail sentences for crimes committed by alcoholics' are favoured over treatment or community-service options (Peele 1987: 207, 208). It might be commented, as Sedgewick (1994: 137) does concerning Szasz, that such thinking 'owes everything to a tropism toward the absolute of punishable free will that itself more than verges on the authoritarian'.

Bunton's discussion (this volume) of 'permissible pleasures' also notes the connection with Puritan thought. But present-day advocates of moderate or controlled drinking as ideology and practice would certainly not define themselves as Puritans. Some indeed tend to try to cast their opposition into the Puritan role. Thus Stanton Peele, who organized a conference on 'permission for pleasure' and co-edited a book from it (Peele and Grant 1999) for an alcohol industry social-aspects organization, in a current discussion lumps together alcohol controls, disease concepts of alcoholism and requirements that authors disclose industry funding as all being modern manifestations in one way or another of 'Temperance ideology' (Peele 2010).

Moral contrasts

There is an obvious conflict between the socioeconomic imperative for alcohol products to be consumed and the increasingly exacting standards of care and attention in present-day societies. The solution to this cultural dilemma has been to place the burden of managing the conflict (and the blame for failure) on the individual. The moderate drinker, who drinks regularly, but without ever becoming intoxicated, is thus a hero of the economic system, painstakingly treading the knife-edge between failure to consume and overconsumption.

Against this positive ideal are set two different versions of the antihero. One is the alcoholic – or the person with alcohol dependence, to use the current technical term. A framing in terms of alcohol dependence points attention to the accumulation of drinking events and troubles over time, and to failure in major social roles – thus one of the DSM-IV criteria for a diagnosis of dependence is that 'important social, occupational or recreational activities are given up or reduced' because of drinking. The intention of the alcoholism movement was that this alcoholism concept would remove responsibility from the drinker, on the premise that a disease formulation would replace a moral framing. But in highly moralized areas, a disease formulation does not do much to remove the moral loading (Room 1983). What the disease formulation does accomplish is to weaken any argument on the necessity of market controls. Public policy on market conditions, it can easily be argued, should not be built around consideration of a small part of the population with a disease condition to which they were predisposed by genetics or upbringing.

The other antihero is perhaps better characterized as a villain – a version of the 'killer drunk' of the anti-drink-driving movement (Gusfield 1984). In this case, the 'loss of control' in question is not about the long-term accumulation of habit. It is rather about self-control as a moment-to-moment expectation – certainly in public spaces, and in many situations in private spaces, too. Intoxication is an obvious threat to this expectation of a civil demeanour and conscious and considered behaviour. The political framing of this antihero is also often in terms of a 'small minority', a few 'rotten apples' who can be dealt with by ASBOs and banning orders.

Putting the blame on the individual level provides a solution to the contradictions of a system built both around expectations of sober attention and around a relatively free availability of alcohol. The solution is congenial to those committed to a free market in alcohol with few or no state controls – including alcohol-beverage industry interests. Thus a recurrent theme of alcohol-industry arguments, as an alternative to market controls, has been 'Why not punish the drunkard?' (Catlin 1931) – or, alternatively, why not provide treatment for the alcoholic? (Fingarette 1988).

But the solutions tend to wear thin around the edges, particularly in terms of how small the minority really is. Almost 4 per cent of US adults qualify for a current alcohol-dependence diagnosis on the basis of their survey responses, and 12.5 per cent qualify on a lifetime basis (Hasin *et al.* 2007). Regular heavy drinkers account for a high proportion of all alcohol consumed; for the US, the top 10 per cent of drinkers account for 55 per cent of all alcohol consumed (Kerr and Greenfield 2007). The proportion of the English population who reported in 2005 drinking more than twice the recommended limit on an occasion[3] on at least one day in the last week was 18 per cent for men and 8 per cent for women (Institute for Alcohol Studies 2009).

Conclusion

The idealization of moderate alcohol consumption and of personal responsibility for controlling drinking behaviour thus becomes a solution for a central contradiction in modern consumer societies. The application of neoliberal ideals of consumer sovereignty, free market access at any hour of the day or night, and unrestrained market promotion tends to push upward the population's alcohol consumption. But in many aspects of daily life – for instance, when at work, when driving a car, when minding children – modern societies require sobriety. The ideological solution to this societal dilemma is to individualize the responsibility for handling it: the onus is on the individual consumer to manage and limit his or her drinking so that it does not interfere with roles requiring sobriety or with public order and domestic peace. The epitome of this ideology is the ideal of the moderate drinker, at the cultural level as a dream to reach for ('continental drinking' in English-speaking and Nordic societies: Olsson 1990; Room 1992) and at the individual level as an ideal of a secular pilgrim's progress.

Notes

1 The AER Centre for Alcohol Policy Research is a joint undertaking of the Alcohol Education and Rehabilitation Foundation, Canberra; the Department of Human Services, Victorian Government; the University of Melbourne, and Turning Point Alcohol and Drug Centre, Fitzroy, Victoria, Australia. This work draws in part on Room (2004b).
2 To a considerable extent, this has been the traditional resolution in the wine cultures of southern Europe. Moving to a 'continental drinking culture' has long been a dream in more northerly European and in English-speaking societies (Chafetz 1967; Olsson 1990), but has largely run up against the stubborn realities of cultural framings of alcohol in which intoxication is valued (Room and Mäkelä 2000).
3 That is, drank more than 64gm of pure alcohol for men, more than 48gm for women.

References

Adler, M. (1991) 'From symbolic exchange to commodity consumption: Anthropological notes on drinking as a symbolic practice', in S. Barrows and R. Room (eds) *Drinking Behavior and Belief in Modern History*, Berkeley: University of California Press, pp. 376–398.

Archibald, H.D. (1990) *The Addiction Research Foundation: A Voyage of Discovery*, Toronto: Addiction Research Foundation.

Babor, T., Caetano, R., Casswell, S., Edwards, G. (2010) *Alcohol – No Ordinary Commodity: Research and Public Policy*, 2nd edn, Oxford: Oxford University Press.

Bell, K., McNaughton, D. and Salmon, A. (2009) 'Medicine, morality and mothering: Public health discourses on foetal alcohol exposure, smoking around children and childhood overnutrition', *Critical Public Health*, 19(2): 155–170.

Bennett, J. (1999) *Ale, Beer, and Brewsters in England: Women's Work in a Changing World, 1300–1600*, New York: Oxford University Press.

Boorman, M. (1999) 'The evolution of impaired driver law – Victoria', paper presented at History of Crime, Policing and Punishment Conference, Canberra, Australia.

Bracken, J. (1955) *Report of the Manitoba Liquor Enquiry Commission*, Winnipeg: The Commission.

Caldwell, P. de H. (1996) 'Whisky-manure engines and "haut, fiery gouts": The Scotch whisky industry and its causal relation to Scotland's economic transformation', *Business and Economic History*, 25(1): 19–26.

Catlin, G.E.G. (1931) *Liquor Control*, New York: Henry Holt.

Chafetz, M. (1967) 'Alcoholism prevention and reality', *Quarterly Journal of Studies on Alcohol*, 28: 345–348.

Citizens for Moderation (1989) 'A Citizens for Moderation brief containing arguments for language modification to the Alcoholic Beverage Labeling Act of 1988', *Journal of Moderation*, 3(5): 1–15.

Consumer Affairs (2007) 'Changes to the Act', *The Grapevine: Liquor Licensing News Bulletin*, Summer: 2.

Courtwright, D.T. (2001) *Forces of Habit: Drugs and the Making of the Modern World*, Cambridge, MA: Harvard University Press.

Crush, J. and Ambler, C. (eds) (1992) *Liquor and Labor in South Africa*, Athens, OH: Ohio University Press.

Duckert, F. (1989) ' "Controlled drinking" – A complicated and contradictory field', in F. Duckert, A. Koski-Jännes and S. Rönnberg (eds) *Perspectives on Controlled Drinking*, Helsinki: Nordic Council for Alcohol and Drug Research, NAD Publication No. 17, pp. 39–54.

Fingarette, H. (1988) *Heavy Drinking: The Myth of Alcoholism as a Disease*, Berkeley: University of California Press.

Graham, J. (1996) *The Secret History of Alcoholism: The Story of Famous Alcoholics and Their Destructive Behavior*, Shaftesbury: Element.

Gusfield, J. (1984) *The Culture of Public Problems: Drinking-Driving and the Symbolic Order*, Chicago: University of Chicago Press.

Gusfield, J. (1991) 'Benevolent repression: Popular culture, social structure and the control of drinking', in S. Barrows and R. Room (eds) *Drinking Behavior and Belief in Modern History*, Berkeley: University of California Press, pp. 399–424.

Harrison, B. (1971) *Drink and the Victorians: The Temperance Question in England 1815–1872*, London: Faber and Faber.

Hasin, D.S., Stinson, F.S., Ogburn, E. and Grant, B.F. (2007) 'Prevalence, correlates, disability, and comorbidity of DSM-IV alcohol abuse and dependence in the United States: Results from the National Epidemiological Survey on Alcohol and Related Conditions', *Archives of General Psychiatry*, 64(7): 830–842.

Houthakker, H.S. and Taylor, L.D. (1970) *Consumer Demand in the United States: Analyses and Projections*, 2nd edn, Cambridge, MA: Harvard University Press.

Institute for Alcohol Studies (2009) 'Drinking in Great Britain', *IAS Fact Sheet*. Online, available at: www.ias.org.uk/resources/factsheets/drinkinggb.pdf (accessed 5 July 2010).

Jellinek, E.M. (1952) 'Phases of alcohol addiction', *Quarterly Journal of Studies on Alcohol*, 13: 673–684.

Kanfer, F.H. (1986) 'Implications of a self-regulation model of therapy for treatment of addictive behaviors', in W.R. Miller and N. Heather (eds) *Treating Addictive Behaviors: Processes of Change*, New York and London: Plenum Press, pp. 29–47.

Kerr, W.C. and Greenfield, T.K. (2007) 'Distribution of alcohol consumption and expenditures and the impact of improved measurement on coverage of alcohol sales in the 2000 National Alcohol Survey', *Alcoholism: Clinical and Experimental Research*, 31(10): 1714–1722.

Levine, H.G. (1985) 'The birth of American alcohol control: Prohibition, the power elite, and the problem of lawlessness', *Contemporary Drug Problems*, 12: 63–115.

Mäkelä, K., Room, R., Single, E., Sulkunen, P. and Walsh, B. (1981) *Alcohol, Society and the State: I. A Comparative Study of Alcohol Control*, Toronto: Addiction Research Foundation.

Mäkelä, P., Rossow, I. and Tryggvesson, K. (2002) 'Who drinks more and less when policies change? The evidence from 50 years of Nordic studies', in R. Room (ed.) *The Effects of Nordic Alcohol Policies: What Happens to Drinking When Alcohol Controls Change?* Helsinki: Nordic Council for Alcohol and Drug Research, NAD Publication 42, pp. 17–70.

Marlatt, G.A. (1985) 'Lifestyle modification', in G.A. Marlatt and J.R. Gordon (eds) *Relapse Prevention: Maintenance Strategies in the Treatment of Addictive Behaviors*, New York: Guilford Press, pp. 280–348.

Mercer, C. (2006) 'Pernod Ricard drinks to carry warning labels', *Beverage Daily*. Online, available at: www.beveragedaily.com/Formulation/Pernod-Ricard-drinks-to-carry-warning-labels (accessed 1 May 2010).

Olsson, B. (1990) 'Alkoholpolitik och alkoholens fenomenologi: Uppfattningar som artikulerats i pressen' ('Alcohol and alcohol's phenomenology: Perceptions that are articulated in the press'), *Alkoholpolitik – Tidskrift för nordisk alkoholforskning*, 7: 184–194.

Peele, S. (1987) 'A moral vision of addiction: How people's values determine whether they become and remain addicts', *Journal of Drug Issues*, 17: 187–215.

Peele, S. (2010) 'Alcohol as evil: Temperance and policy', *Addiction Research and Theory*, 18(19): 379–382.

Peele, S. and Grant, M. (eds) (1999) *Alcohol and Pleasure: A Health Perspective*, International Center for Alcohol Policies, Series on Alcohol in Society, Philadelphia: Brunner/Maazel.

Room, R. (1983) 'Sociological aspects of the disease concept of alcoholism', in R. Smart, F.B. Glaser, Y. Israel, H. Kalant, R.E. Popham and W.E. Schmidt (eds) *Research Advances in Alcohol and Drug Problems*, vol. 7, New York: Plenum, pp. 47–91.

Room, R. (1984a) 'Alcohol control and public health', *Annual Review of Public Health*, 5: 293–317.

Room, R. (1984b) 'A "reverence for strong drink": The lost generation and the elevation of alcohol in American culture', *Journal of Studies on Alcohol*, 45: 540–546.

Room, R. (1992) 'The impossible dream? Routes to reducing alcohol problems in a temperance culture', *Journal of Substance Abuse*, 4: 91–106.

Room, R. (2004a) 'Alcohol and harm reduction, then and now', *Critical Public Health*, 14: 329–344.

Room, R. (2004b) 'Controlled drinking as a moral achievement and a social program', in H. Klingemann, R. Room, H. Rosenberg, S. Schatzmann, L. Sobell and M. Sobell (eds) *Kontrolliertes Trinken als Behandlungsziel – Bestandesaufnahme des aktuellen Wissens (Controlled Drinking as a Treatment Goal – An Inventory of Current Knowledge)*, Bern: Institut für Sozialplanung und Sozialmanagement, Hochschule für Sozialarbeit, pp. 148–157.

Room, R. (2004c) 'Disabling the public interest: Alcohol policies and strategies for England', *Addiction*, 99: 1083–1089.

Room, R. (2010) 'The long reaction against the wowser: The prehistory of alcohol deregulation in Australia', *Health Sociology Review*, 19(2): 151–163.

Room, R. and Mäkelä, K. (2000) 'Typologies of the cultural position of drinking', *Journal of Studies on Alcohol*, 61: 475–483.

Room, R., Jernigan, D., Carlini-Cotrim, B., Gureje, O., Mäkelä, K., Marshall, M., Medina-Mora, M.E., Monteiro, M., Parry, C., Partanen, J., Riley, L. and Saxena, S. (2002) *Alcohol in Developing Societies: A Public Health Approach*, Helsinki: Finnish Foundation for Alcohol Studies.

Room, R., Stoduto, G., Demers, A., Ogborne, A. and Giesbrecht, N. (2006) 'Alcohol in the Canadian context', in N. Giesbrecht, A. Demers, A. Ogborne, R. Room, G. Stoduto and E. Lindquist (eds) *Sober Reflections: Commerce, Public Health, and the Evolution of Alcohol Policy in Canada, 1980–2000*, Montreal and Kingston: McGill-Queen's University Press, pp. 14–42.

Rosenzweig, R. (1983) *Eight Hours for What We Will: Workers and Leisure in an Industrial City, 1870–1920*, New York: Oxford University Press.

Rubin, J.L. (1979) 'Shifting perspectives on the alcoholism treatment movement 1940–1955', *Journal of Studies on Alcohol*, 40: 376–386.

Rumbarger, J.J. (1989) *Profits, Power, and Prohibition: Alcohol Reform and the Industrializing of America, 1800–1930*, Albany: State University of New York Press.

Sedgewick, E.K. (1994) *Tendencies*, London: Routledge.

Stockwell, T. (1986) 'Cracking an old chestnut: Is controlled drinking possible for the person who has been severely alcohol dependent?', *British Journal of Addiction*, 81: 455–456.

Stockwell, T.R., Single, E., Hawks, D.V. and Rehm, J. (1997) 'Sharpening the focus of alcohol policy from aggregate consumption to harm and risk reduction', *Addiction Research*, 5(1): 1–9.

Sutton, C. (1998) *Swedish Alcohol Discourse: Constructions of a Social Problem*, Uppsala: Uppsala University Library, Studia Sociologica Upsaliensia, 45.

Wilkinson, C. (2008) 'Public discourse on the revised Australian Alcohol Guidelines for Low-Risk Drinking', (Australasian Professional Society on Alcohol and Drugs), Sydney, Australia.

4 Between alarmists and sceptics
On the cultural politics of obesity scholarship and public policy

Michael Gard

Introduction

While moral and medical anxiety about fatness seems to have fluctuated over time and space, a number of important historical works suggest that it increased and mutated in Western countries during the last 120 years or so (Schwartz 1986; Stearns 1997). The emergence of the 'obesity epidemic' around the turn of the twenty-first century (Gard 2011), then, was in many ways simply the latest instalment in an ongoing cultural and scientific dialogue about health and the body.

And yet, today's 'obesity epidemic' is also a distinct historical event. For example, as an idea the 'obesity epidemic' harnesses the relatively recent and growing influence of risk-factor medicine and epidemiology, scientific traditions that are premised on seeking out the underlying causes of disease in order to cure or, better still, pre-emptively prevent it. Epidemiologists, in particular, were instrumental in bringing recent rises in Western body weights to global attention and is the discipline most concerned with trying to quantify healthy body weight and how much of a risk being 'too heavy' really is.

A detailed history of the twenty-first century's 'obesity epidemic' is not yet written, but it does appear that epidemiology was joined by advocates from a wide range of fields, including public health and mainstream medicine, to announce that a health crisis was upon us, a crisis that would lead to declining life expectancy, an explosion in chronic disease and the collapse of health systems across the Western world (see Gard and Wright 2005; Gard 2011 for a summary and an analysis of these claims). Perhaps inevitably, the rhetoric of 'crisis' and 'epidemic' was quickly engaged by oppositional and sceptical voices. While alarmists have characterized the 'obesity epidemic' as a looming global health catastrophe, sceptics have argued that the consequences of rising obesity levels have either been greatly exaggerated or are unclear (e.g. Gard and Wright 2001; Campos 2004; Oliver 2006).

While my own position as an obesity sceptic has been articulated in previous publications (especially Gard and Wright 2001, 2005), more recently

I have drawn on my role as one of the combatants in the 'obesity wars' to construct a kind of anatomy of the obesity controversy, such as it is. In passing, I would not want to over-emphasize the degree to which there has actually been a debate between obesity alarmists and sceptics. After all, the obesity alarmist camp includes the vast majority of the medical and epidemiological research communities. The overwhelming dominance of alarmists means that, for the most part, sceptics have simply been ignored. There are signs that this situation is changing slightly, but it remains the case that most alarmists simply do not see the need to debate sceptics.

In this chapter I want to move beyond the idea of there being two camps in debates about obesity. There certainly are two broad groupings, but I want to provide a more complex account of the different groups that make up both sides. For example, on the alarmist side there are those who favour ramping up the stigmatization of individuals in order to fight obesity; a shame-led public-health agenda, as it were (see McCullough, this volume, for a discussion of parallels in the tobacco field). Other alarmists come in more socially democratic hues, emphasizing broadly focused social policies and legislation.

However, my own side, the sceptics, is perhaps more interesting. Obesity sceptics are made up of a kaleidoscope of interest groups with different and sometimes diametrically opposed political leanings. They include feminists, queer theorists, libertarians, far-right-wing conspiracy types and New Ageists. We are, to say the least, a motley crew.

My purpose here is to ask some familiar but important questions: *why* do we believe and advocate for the things we do? More specifically, *how* do we organize and use 'evidence' to suit our own ideological and, particularly with respect to academic scholarship, theoretical commitments? What, actually, does it mean to 'weigh up the evidence'? These are questions I am inclined to ask of both myself and others, and to wonder whether asking these questions might cause us to think or act differently. And if we are not changed by these questions, why not? In other words, I am wrestling not only with the substance of belief – what and why do we believe? – but also with what we might call the ethics of belief – how should we believe?

The alarmists

From a purely academic point of view, it is worth considering the range of alarmists' positions because, as I will show later in this chapter, sceptics often assume alarmists to operate from a single base motive. This assumption is rhetorically convenient but, because of their generalizing gloss, the arguments of sceptics are often easily dismissed by alarmists and, I think, harm the reputation of critical health scholarship.

I will spend less time discussing obesity alarmism because, for most readers, the arguments they put forward will be well-known. What is instructive, though, is the different forms of argumentation used by alarmists to explain or, in some cases, suggest cures for the 'obesity epidemic'. For example, many readers will be aware of the standard set of propositions that characterize both academic and popular comment: rising obesity levels are the product of changing lifestyles that make physical exertion less necessary and high-calorie food more palatable and available than in the past. In the academic literature we read: 'Obesity is the most obvious manifestation of the global epidemic of sedentary lifestyles and excessive energy intake' (Cameron *et al.* 2003: 427). Meanwhile, with particular attention to children, the popular media regularly 'reports' that children 'spend a lot of time playing computer games, watching television, and eating fatty snacks like chips and chocolate, instead of playing outside and eating nutritious meals' (Head 2003: n.p.).

I have discussed elsewhere the confused and contradictory state of the obesity science literature, particularly when it comes to explaining the causes of increasing obesity (Gard and Wright 2005). Is it food or physical activity? Car ownership or televisions and computers? The amount or types of food we eat? However, if we look more broadly, pooling academic and non-academic commentators together, we can see that a range of other tensions exists. In terms of cultural politics, perhaps the most obvious of these tensions centres on the issue of personal culpability. As LeBesco and McNaughton (this volume) also note, there is no shortage of commentators, both inside and outside the obesity research community, who argue that individuals are to blame for allowing themselves to become obese. Researchers focus on individuals in two ways. First, they do this directly by simply saying or writing that individuals are to blame. This ranges from leading lights in the field describing the entire American population as 'physical activity sluggards' (Lee and Paffenbarger 1996: 206) to, more recently, a group of Australian researchers who blamed childhood obesity on parents being 'bad role models' (Wood 2005: 9). A recent recipient of the Canadian Obesity Network's outstanding thesis competition proposed that parents were morally obligated to prevent their children from becoming obese and that there are potential legal implications for parents who fail to live up to their obligations (Canadian Obesity Network 2006).

Second, researchers blame individuals indirectly by focusing their research and public statements on personal behaviours. For example, Chakravarthy and Booth (2003) write about an 'epidemic' of inactivity as though people simply wake up and decide to be inactive, and there is now an entire epidemiological sub-discipline devoted to explaining the 'determinants' of the physical-activity behaviour of individuals (see Gard 2008 for a discussion of this field's preoccupation with modifying individual behaviour).

But while, as we will see in this chapter, there are obesity sceptics who say that the idea of an 'obesity epidemic' is, per se, an individualizing discourse, there are alarmists who make the opposite argument; that focusing on obesity alerts us to the social and structural determinants of body weight and health. For example, Ludwig (2007: 2326) argues:

> Parents must take responsibility for their children's welfare by providing high-quality food, limiting television viewing, and modeling a healthful lifestyle. But why should Mr. and Ms. G.'s efforts to protect their children from life-threatening illness be undermined by massive marketing campaigns from the manufacturers of junk food? Why are their children subjected to the temptation of such food in the school cafeteria and vending machines? Why don't they have the opportunity to exercise their bodies during the school day?

If anything, Budd and Hayman (2008: 111) are more direct: 'Addressing the obesity crisis requires a paradigm shift away from blaming individuals for the lack of willpower to control their eating and physical activity to one of recognizing the "toxic" or "obesogenic" environment as a primary determinant.'

Of course, arguing for a 'paradigm shift' to change our 'toxic' environment means changing the way we should live or be allowed to live. Many obesity researchers talk about 'making healthy choices the easy choices', a rhetorical move that, to some extent, obscures the fact that re-engineering people's everyday lives to make them exercise more and eat less requires tough decisions that will not please everybody. Thus, diametrically opposed to those who would emphasize individual responsibility are researchers who say that, in the end, the war on obesity will only be won through strong, decisive, centralized decision-making, the kind that is usually the preserve of governments. Swinburn (2008), for example, argues that the 'obesity epidemic' is an example of business success but market failure and, as such, is a classic case for strong government intervention. In his view, what is needed is a strong policy 'spine' of 'hard paternalism' accompanied with the 'soft paternalism' of health promotion. He also thinks that 'stealth' interventions that piggy-back along with efforts to reduce CO_2 emissions, city congestion and other problems will probably also improve the obesity situation.

What emerges here is a kind of fantasy that is actually quite common in the obesity-research literature: the fantasy of a social policy context in which every arm of government is synergistically involved in the war on obesity. But note also here that Swinburn feels that the obesity epidemic represents, in part, the failure of capitalism to produce sound health outcomes. Strong governments, not market forces, are the only hope.

The idea that the 'obesity epidemic' is a sign of the failure of capitalism has been made a number of times in the media. Commentators who take this line usually also emphasize the extent to which poor Westerners are more likely to be affected by obesity than rich Westerners (e.g. Hutton 2002; Krugman 2005). This is interesting because, as we will shortly see, there are some obesity writers who think that the 'obesity epidemic' can be blamed, not on capitalism, but its enemies.

The empirical sceptics

The idea of an 'obesity epidemic' or crisis has provoked a varied set of oppositional responses, and these could be analysed and categorized in many different ways. The analysis that I offer below is simply one amongst these possibilities, albeit one that strikes me as particularly instructive.

First, there is a group of writers who have refuted the idea of an obesity epidemic by engaging more or less directly with the original obesity research literature (e.g. Campos 2004; Basham *et al*. 2006; Oliver 2006). These critiques have emerged almost exclusively from outside the scientific/ epidemiological obesity research community. While I contrast this group of writers with what, in the next section, I call 'ideological sceptics', I do not want to suggest that the authors I discuss in this section do not have ideological allegiances. They clearly do. However, I use the term 'empirical sceptics' to group together those writers who at least claim to base their obesity scepticism on *their own* assessment of 'the evidence' rather than relying on the assessment of others. That is, my sense is that 'empirical sceptics' *represent themselves* as having based their conclusions purely on the scientific evidence.

Empirical sceptics have attempted to make the argument that an objective treatment of the research literature shows that alarmist claims are wrong or exaggerated. That is, they claim to be the true and unbiased voice of science. Three obvious examples can be found in Gaesser's (2002) *Big Fat Lies: The Truth About Your Weight and Your Health*, Campos's (2004) *The Obesity Myth: Why America's Obsession with Weight is Hazardous to Your Health*, and Oliver's (2006) *Fat Politics: The Real Story Behind America's Obesity Epidemic*. The importance of claiming the mantle of truth is clearly important in the titles of each of these publications. Likewise, each has a similar take on the 'obesity epidemic': it is more or less a conspiracy in the obesity-research community, the product of poor science, economic self-interest and stubbornness in the face of overwhelming contrary evidence. Campos (2004: 13), for example, continually asserts that 'anyone who bothers to examine the evidence' will agree with his conclusion that obesity has been over-hyped.

The politics of these writers is not always abundantly clear, although each tends to represent themselves as working against obesity as a moral panic and the demonization of overweight and obese people. They also tend to be critical of the actions of corporations, particularly those that sponsor research into weight-loss drugs as well as those that make, market and sell junk food. Although political labels are tricky here, they probably represent the social-democratic, conventionally left-liberal end of obesity scepticism, concerning themselves with the way powerful groups, such as ivy-league universities, multi-national corporations and government health authorities, are making life difficult for the less powerful majority of society.

Taking us in a different direction, the edited volume *Panic Nation: Unpicking the Myths We're Told About Food and Health* (Feldman and Marks 2005) is a collection of short myth-busting essays, covering a wide range of subjects including exercise, healthy-eating and obesity. There is an unmistakable ideological agenda running through *Panic Nation* that science is a truth machine and that the existence of untruths is the fault of forces either ignorant of, or openly hostile to, the techniques of proper science. In his chapter on exercise and sports, Aichroth (2005) argues that excessive exercise causes a great deal of injury and costs nations a lot of money. He also writes that exercise, except in extreme cases, does not have much effect on obesity since most energy is burned through maintaining body temperature. Aichroth's villains are what he calls the sports lobby and exercise 'nuts', both of whom he dismisses as having tried to foist their own fanaticisms on the rest of us: 'The simplest aerobic exercise is walking. Half an hour of brisk walking every day will provide sufficient aerobic exercise to offset any health disadvantage due to a sedentary lifestyle' (Aichroth 2005: 267).

Likewise, Marks' (2005: 59) chapter on obesity rails against 'single-issue pressure groups' for not understanding the statistical risks of fatness and, he claims, unfairly targeting the makers of so-called junk food. As with most of the chapters of *Panic Nation*, the war for the truth about health is seen as being fought between, on the side for good, mainstream medicine and, on the side of scientific ignorance, New-Agers, feminists and a collection of anti-capitalists.

On the whole, the tone of *Panic Nation* is conservative and curmudgeonly, proudly so in my reading of it. However, perhaps the dominant form of 'empirical scepticism' comes from a group of writers whose cultural and political affiliations are less ambiguous.

Writing for the libertarian and avowedly free-market think tank The Fraser Institute, Esmail and Brown (2005) articulate a particularly virulent form of the idea that, rather than being victims, overweight and obese people are a burden on society. Esmail and Brown are uncomfortable with anti-obesity social policies that, they claim, infringe on people's freedoms, especially since their assessment is that obesity is not such a big problem. But:

> If governments decide to act, however, the best way to account for the costs the obese impose on society is to require these individuals to bear those costs that result from their decisions. This could be as simple as introducing health premiums scaled by the cost that individual's lifestyle choices imposes on others. A scaled premium not only solves the problem of an increased burden on all Canadians created by the few

who may be able to choose otherwise, but also gives those who are obese a reason to lose the extra pounds.

(n.p.)

A number of other examples of the libertarian strain in obesity scepticism could be offered. One that garnered some media attention is Basham *et al.*'s (2006) *Diet Nation: Exposing the Obesity Crusade*. As with some other empirical sceptics, we see in the title of their work the idea that they, the authors, will 'expose' the truth about obesity where mainstream obesity science has failed. In other words, in my view what is important for empirical sceptics is not so much that their treatment of the scientific evidence is superior to anyone else's, but rather that they *represent* themselves as the voice of hard-headed scientific sobriety (see also Social Issues Research Centre 2005).

It is interesting in the context of a discussion of cultural politics that neither the text of *Diet Nation* nor the publicity around the book high-lighted the political affiliations of the authors. Basham, in particular, is an active member of free-market think tanks the Cato Institute and the Democracy Institute. He, too, like Esmail and Brown (2005), is connected to and writes for the Fraser Institute. It is therefore no coincidence that *Diet Nation* also blames the obesity epidemic on the enemies of capitalism, going even as far as suggesting that the obesity 'crusaders' are actually socialists in disguise. All this should remind us that, regardless of the overall political thrust of their arguments, it is extremely rare for alarmists or, for that matter, sceptics to make their political affiliations clear.

This form of free-market libertarian obesity scepticism is widespread and a number of newspaper and magazine columnists take their lead from it (e.g. Duffy 2007; Lyons 2007). It has also been popular on far-right-wing, pro-gun, pro-American websites where the idea that obesity alarm-ists are nanny-state communists who simply want to stop us from having fun plays well (e.g. Political Correctness Watch 2005).

The ideological sceptics

For better or worse, being part of a clan of one sort or another is an almost inevitable dimension of academic life. For over ten years I have been men-tored within a research community that (mostly for the better) is strongly marked by the influence of feminism, post-structuralism and the various strands of what is sometimes called 'critical social science'. In my own field of physical education, like most others, there are areas of disagreement and debate and individual scholars who work independently of the clans. Nonetheless, I now want to offer a sense of the way a certain kind of obesity scepticism has become the default position for some academics. I offer this more as food for thought than full-frontal critique; my purpose here is simply to work against the tendency in all academic fields of study towards ossifying orthodoxies.

Because space prevents me from a more detailed explanation, in what follows I will rely on what I hope are at least defensible short-hands. To this end, my proposition in this section is that ideological scepticism emerges out of two distinct but related sets of received ideas that guide and shape the kinds of arguments ideological sceptics are inclined to make.

First, ideological scepticism is steeped in the feminist critique of science. It hardly needs to be stressed that I am glossing a vast and diverse literature here and that there is no single feminist critique of science, and nothing approaching a unified core set of positions and arguments. However, I think we can say that the feminist critique has provided intellectual ballast for a number of widely used ideas – ideas that, in turn, have become characteristic of this intellectual movement: for example, science's preoccupation with numbers and quantification, the fantasy of objectivity, the privileging of whiteness over non-whiteness, Western over non-Western, male over female, 'man' over 'nature', order over perversity, and reason over emotion, have all been the targets of feminist analysis. Taken together, they provide scholars with a set of ideas and methods for seeing, interpreting and critiquing science.

My second assertion in this section is that ideological sceptics have drawn from the critique of neoliberalism, once again a huge body of diverse scholarship. Owing much to Foucauldian analyses of language, power and governmentality, the critique of neoliberalism tends to emphasize the dominance of free-market ideas, the application of (often crude) scientific rationality to social policy, increasing governmental and institutional interest in people's 'personal' conduct, and the influence of notions of individual responsibility and performative morality on identity construction (Howell and Ingham 2001; McGregor 2001). Western neoliberal citizens are, for better and worse, enmeshed in a system that, despite (or perhaps because of) increasing cultural, ethnic and economic diversity, believes that rational, scientific solutions are possible to all the problems and dilemmas we face. But more than this, the critique of neoliberalism is interested in the way new codes of morality are being produced in an attempt to discipline people's desires, behaviours, relationships and subjectivities.

I accept that there will be some readers who are dissatisfied with one or both of my theoretical short-hands here. For those prepared to persevere, I want to propose further that there are obvious synergies between the feminist critique of science and the critique of neoliberalism. For example, both draw our attention to what we might call naive-scientism; the ideological preference for scientific solutions in situations where they may not be appropriate or ethical. In addition, both want us to think about the individuals and groups who are the intended and unintended casualties of scientistic, neoliberal rationalities.

Not all ideological sceptics draw equally on these two sets of ideas. For example, Robison and Carrier (2004), advocates for *Health at Every Size* –

a movement with grass-roots and academic followers that campaigns against dieting and in favour of body-weight acceptance – argue that the 'obesity epidemic' is essentially an extension of patriarchal science's centuries-old persecution of women. In their book *The Spirit and Science of Holistic Health* (2004: 228, emphasis added), they write:

> Traditional weight management approaches, *like all other aspects of Western health care*, emanate from the biomedical, reductionist paradigm, which is rooted in patriarchy and the oppression of women. On the surface it may look as though efforts to control body weight are simply based on a desire to make people 'healthier.' On closer examination, however, the disparate social emphasis on women regarding thinness, the emphasis on control over the body, and even the subtle messages that higher moral standing is obtained through starving and denial of pleasurable eating are all perspectives that run directly parallel to the values of Epoch II and the Scientific Revolution.

Notice here the totalizing spirit that seems to run through phrases such as 'like all other aspects of Western health care'. In other words, all forms of medicine and healthcare apparently stem from the intended or unintended oppression of women. Rather than strange or novel, within this explanatory framework the idea of an 'obesity epidemic' is little more than a symptom of a cultural sickness that goes back to the birth of Western rationality. For Robison and Carrier, there is no way out; despite good intentions, all manifestations of modern scientific medicine will be washed away in the coming 'holistic health' revolution or, as they call it, 'Epoch III'.

Far less extreme is the work of scholars such as Schwartz (1986), Ritenbaugh (1982), Jutel (2001, 2009), and Jutel and Buetow (2007) who have described the course of body-weight science over recent centuries. However, the issue of whether the past explains the present or the present explains this past is surely in play here. If we take it for granted that health researchers and authorities are particularly exercised about people's body weights today, do we understand this by looking back in history to see where medical concern about body weight began and then project that forward as the cause of today's anxieties (the past explains the present)? Or, rather, is it possible that what these historians have done is to begin with a social phenomenon to explain – the 'obesity epidemic' – and then simply arranged certain historical events into the kind of narrative about medical science they always wanted to tell (the present explains the past)? Jutel (2001: 283), for example, asks us to accept that modern concerns about obesity are the historical legacy of medical science's quest to quantify, manipulate and control the human body:

> In this paper, I argue that an attraction to quantification and a belief that appearance mirrors the 'true' inner self, compounded by a

religious fascination in establishing rules of normality, underpins a medical and cultural over-reliance on weight as an indicator of health. The lean, spare body is a 'good body,' evidence of strong moral fiber, of someone who, constantly vigilant, 'looks after themselves.' I will explore how such beliefs are crystallized in contemporary health policies.

In this passage we can see the influence of the feminist critique's mistrust of numbers and quantification as well as the critique of neoliberalism's concern with the disciplining of human bodies through institutional apparatuses and performative morality. As an obesity sceptic, Jutel believes that modern medicine is 'over-reliant' on body weight and wants us to understand this not as a spontaneous sign of medicine's care for human health and the preservation of life, but as a kind of Freudian hang-up; a kind of obsession that gets in the way of it treating human body weight more rationally and ethically. Elsewhere, Jutel (2009) assumes that we can take it as read that the scientific evidence alone does not warrant the current level of concern about obesity. Instead, we must look for other motives.

We see a similar kind of rhetorical move in Monaghan's (2008) *Men and the War on Obesity: A Sociological Study*, except in this case the charge of malign intentions is made more explicitly: 'I would maintain that the institutionalized attack on fat is really about bodily regulation, morality and other sociological concerns (e.g. individualizing and de-politicizing healthism, the expansion of markets) rather than actually promoting biomedical health in the population' (2008: 70).

Like Jutel, Monaghan argues that medical concern about obesity is not, at base, a concern with health at all and that those who prosecute the 'attack on fat' are, at best, suffering from a form of false consciousness. But Monaghan goes further. He also suggests that the war on obesity is 'really about' holding individuals responsible for their own health ('individualizing' and 'de-politicizing'), thus, I take him to mean, failing to address the social and structural causes of ill-health. This is interesting because, as we saw above, there are many obesity researchers who argue in favour of fighting obesity precisely on the grounds of addressing health inequalities, and that addressing obesity draws greater, not less, attention to health inequalities.

This is clearly not an argument likely to impress Halse (2009) who, like Monaghan, smells a conspiracy in all this talk of obesity and the Body Mass Index (BMI):

Because governments and their agents have committed intense political energy and considerable financial resources to constructing the biocitizen, the virtue discourse of a normative BMI is not an innocent bystander in choreographing the future. But what has been buried in the jetsam and flotsam of its wake are bigger, more difficult issues: hunger; poverty; physical abuse; lack of fresh water, medical care and education; discrimination and inequalities; social and economic disadvantage. A cynic might wonder if this is a stratagem – a bio-political ruse – by governments and their agents to deflect the citizenry's attention from the social justice issues that continue to blight the lives of individuals and the well-being of communities and nations.

(2009: 57)

Whether or not a statement of this kind is made with tongue in cheek, as I think it was, it is interesting to note how the resistance to social control, articulated in this form of left-of-centre academic scepticism, echoes the concerns made by right-of-centre libertarian sceptics; both are concerned about intervention in our lives but, for the former, the worry is that excessive focus on obesity makes us forget about the structural determinants of health while, for the latter, it is our personal liberties that are at stake.

Strange bedfellows

In the hands of different sceptics, the 'obesity epidemic' emerges as both an attack on capitalism *as well as* the triumph of neoliberal thinking, both a perversion of proper science and the embodiment of its deepest traditions. While some see it as symptomatic of a lamentable flight from individual moral responsibility, others see it as a mean-spirited and moralistic attack on the poor and marginal. For writers like Jutel, it is driven in part by a preoccupation with numbers, while Marks thinks it betrays an ignorance of them. But the same is true for the alarmist camp. While there are many obesity researchers who argue that a focus on individual responsibility is futile, the vast majority of obesity-intervention research seeks to change the behaviour of individuals. It is also not difficult to find free-market alarmists who completely reject the idea of corporate responsibility and appear convinced that the only cure for obesity is a rejection of post-1960s moral liberalism and a return to family values and personal self-control (Fumento 1997).

Taking all the writers I have discussed together, what I see is that it is possible both to reach the same conclusion given diametrically opposed starting points, but also to start with the same assumptions only to arrive at opposite conclusions. There are surely grounds here to wonder if both the starting points *and* the conclusions that people reach are not in some important sense arbitrary or, conversely, predetermined. Put another way, are the theories we use and the conclusions we reach better understood as part of a self-styling process? Are they more about a desire to be a certain kind of person or belong to a particular group? Is it possible to escape group-think or the tyranny of our pet theories?

Turning to my own interests in critical public-health scholarship, my view is that we spend too little time considering our theoretical alternatives or engaging in comparative theoretical work. At the very least, in the examples I have offered in this chapter, it is difficult to tell whether theoretical or political allegiances have simply determined the position taken by the author, or whether these allegiances are completely inconsequential; both situations are possible. Either way, these are, for me, both somewhat startling and unsettling conclusions, particularly given that I cling to some hope that the things I advocate for and against are driven by more than either – or both – sheer whim and blind obedience. Perhaps the more important question is how to tell the difference between the two. Perhaps what is required is a more robust and personally frank account of the way moral, ideological and theoretical motivations intersect, coalesce and blur. Put more simply, what seems at stake for me is a clearer explanation of what it means to be rational.

References

Aichroth, P. (2005) 'Exercise and sports', in S. Feldman and V. Marks (eds) *Panic Nation: Unpicking the Myths We're Told About Food and Health*, London: John Blake, pp. 261–268.

Basham, P., Gori, G. and Luik, J. (2006) *Diet Nation: Exposing the Obesity Crusade*, London: The Social Affairs Unit.

Budd, G.M. and Hayman, L.L. (2008) 'Addressing the childhood obesity crisis: A call to action', *American Journal of Maternal Child Nursing*, 33(2): 111–118.

Cameron, A.J., Welborn, T.A., Zimmet, P.Z., Dunstan, D.W., Owen, N., Salmon, J., Dalton, M., Jolley, D. and Shaw, J.E. (2003) 'Overweight and obesity in Australia: The 1999–2000 Australian Diabetes, Obesity and Lifestyle Study (AusDiab)', *Medical Journal of Australia*, 178(9): 427–432.

Campos, P. (2004) *The Obesity Myth: Why America's Obsession with Weight is Hazardous to Your Health*, New York: Gotham Books.

Canadian Obesity Network (2006) 'Are parents morally obligated to prevent obesity in their children?' Canada Obesity Network. Online, available at: www.obesitynetwork.ca/detail.aspx?dt=1336&pp=&cat1=181&tp=18&lk=yes (accessed 22 September 2006).

Chakravarthy, M.V. and Booth, F.W. (2003) 'Inactivity and inaction: We can't afford either', *Archives of Pediatrics and Adolescent Medicine*, 157(8): 731–732.

Duffy, M. (2007) 'Don't fall for the big fat lie when proof of the padding is thin', *Sydney Morning Herald*, 15 December: 31.

Esmail, N. and Brown, J. (2005) 'The wrong defense for tackling obesity', *The Fraser Institute*. Online, available at: www.fraserinstitute.ca/shared/readmore1.asp?sNav=ed&id=352 (accessed 3 November 2005).

Feldman, S. and Marks, V. (eds) (2005) *Panic Nation: Unpicking the Myths We're Told About Food and Health*, London: John Blake.

Fumento, M. (1997) *The Fat of the Land: The Obesity Epidemic and How Overweight Americans Can Help Themselves*, New York: Viking.

Gaesser, G.A. (2002) *Big Fat Lies: The Truth About Your Weight and Your Health*, Carlsbad: Gurze Books.

Gard, M. (2008) ' "Couch potatoes" and "wind-up dolls"? A critical assessment of the ethics of youth physical activity research', in A.L. Smith and S.J.H. Biddle (eds) *Youth Physical Activity and Sedentary Behaviour: Challenges and Solutions*, Champaign: Human Kinetics, pp. 115–138.

Gard, M. (2011) *The End of the Obesity Epidemic*, London: Routledge, forthcoming.

Gard, M. and Wright, J. (2001) 'Managing uncertainty: Obesity discourses and physical education in a risk society', *Studies in Philosophy and Education*, 20(6): 535–549.

Gard, M. and Wright, J. (2005) *The Obesity Epidemic: Science, Morality and Ideology*, London: Routledge.

Halse, C. (2009) 'Bio-citizenship: Virtue discourses and the birth of the bio-citizen', in J. Wright and V. Harwood (eds) *Biopolitics and the 'Obesity Epidemic': Governing Bodies*, New York: Routledge, pp. 45–59.

Head, J. (2003) 'Fighting fat kids: fat chance?', *ABC Online*. Online, available at: www.abc.net.au/health/regions/features/fightingfatkids/default.htm (accessed 1 October 2003).

Howell, J. and Ingham, A. (2001) 'From social problem to personal issue: The language of lifestyle', *Cultural Studies*, 15(2): 326–351.

Hutton, W. (2002) 'Fat is a capitalist issue', *Observer*, 27 January: 30.

Jutel, A. (2001) 'Does size really matter? Weight and values in public health', *Perspectives in Biology and Medicine*, 44(2): 283–296.

Jutel, A. (2009) 'Doctor's orders: Diagnosis, medical authority and the exploitation of the fat body', in J. Wright and V. Harwood (eds) *Biopolitics and the 'Obesity Epidemic': Governing Bodies*, New York: Routledge: 60–77.

Jutel, A. and Buetow, S. (2007) 'A picture of health? Unmasking the role of appearance in health', *Perspectives in Biology and Medicine*, 50(3): 421–434.

Krugman, P. (2005) 'Girth of a nation', *New York Times*, 4 July: 13.

Lee, I.M. and Paffenbarger, R.S. (1996) 'How much physical activity is optimal for health? Methodological considerations', *Research Quarterly for Exercise and Sport*, 67(2): 206–208.

Ludwig, D.S. (2007) 'Childhood obesity – the shape of things to come', *New England Journal of Medicine*, 357(23): 2325–2327.

Lyons, R. (2007) 'The war on obesity is a war on the poor', *Spiked Online*. Online, available at: www.spiked-online.com/index.php?/site/article/3674/ (accessed 28 November).

McGregor, S. (2001) 'Neoliberalism and health care', *International Journal of Consumer Studies*, 25(2): 82–89.

Marks, V. (2005) 'Obesity', in S. Feldman and V. Marks (eds) *Panic Nation: Unpicking the Myths We're Told About Food and Health*, London: John Blake, pp. 53–60.

Monaghan, L.F. (2008) *Men and the War on Obesity: A Sociological Study*, London: Routledge.

Oliver, J.E. (2006) *Fat Politics: The Real Story Behind America's Obesity Epidemic*, Oxford: Oxford University Press.

Political Correctness Watch (2005) *Fat and Fiction*. Online, available at: http://pcwatch.blogspot.com/2005_06_01_archive.html (accessed 11 March 2008).

Ritenbaugh, C. (1982) 'Obesity as a culture-bound syndrome', *Culture, Medicine and Psychiatry*, 6(4): 347–361.

Robison, J. and Carrier, K. (2004) *The Spirit and Science of Holistic Health*, Bloomington: AuthorHouse.

Schwartz, H. (1986) *Never Satisfied: A Cultural History of Diets, Fantasies and Fat*, New York: Free Press.

Social Issues Research Centre (2005) *Obesity and the Facts: An Analysis of Data from the Health Survey for England 2003*, Oxford: Social Issues Research Centre.

Stearns, P.N. (1997) *Fat History: Bodies and Beauty in the Modern West*, New York: New York University Press.

Swinburn, B.A. (2008) 'Obesity prevention: The role of policies, laws and regulations', *Australia and New Zealand Health Policy*, 5(12), doi:10.1186/1743–8462–5–12.

Wood, M. (2005) 'Parents to blame for obese children', *The Sun-Herald*, 13 February: 9.

5 Legislating abjection?

Second-hand smoke, tobacco-control policy and the public's health

Kirsten Bell

Introduction

Since the 1990s, tobacco-control policy has been characterized by an over-whelming focus on the dangers of second-hand smoke and the need to protect the public from this health 'risk'. Smoke-free legislation has been implemented in an unprecedented number of countries, and provinces and states across the USA, Canada and Australia have also enacted comprehensive indoor smoking bans in public places. Even countries historically considered to be highly resistant to such legislation (e.g. France) have recently begun to follow suit.

The widespread implementation of indoor smoking bans since the turn of the twenty-first century has been followed by growing calls to enact outdoor smoking bans in public places (e.g. Bloch and Shopland 2000; Repace 2000; Thomson *et al.* 2008; Walsh *et al.* 2008). For example, at the time of writing, smoking bans have been proposed for Vancouver beaches, and the neighbouring city of White Rock has already enacted a smoking ban at any outdoor gathering place, including parks, sports fields, playgrounds, beaches, etc. (City of White Rock 2008). Other initiatives of note include efforts to ban smoking in quasi-private spaces such as cars carrying children (Vergakis 2006; *The Age* 2007; Canadian Press 2007) and apartment buildings (Kline 2000; CACBC 2008).

Such moves speak to the extraordinary transformation in public health and popular attitudes towards smoking over the past two decades, which has been recast from a socially acceptable practice into an intrinsically dangerous, irresponsible and selfish one. Key to the present vilification of smoking is the assumption that smokers harm not only themselves but also *put others at risk* via the polluting and dangerous second-hand smoke they expel from their bodies.

In this chapter, I am interested in exploring the cultural context of second-hand smoke as a public-health issue. However, this is a task that has become increasingly delicate in the politically charged environment of tobacco research, where examinations that de-centre the 'truth' of scientific scholarship on second-hand smoke are immediately open to attack from the tobacco-control community. As Sullum (1998: xiii) notes, 'anti-smoking activists and their allies have portrayed criticism of the case against secondhand smoke as a tobacco industry plot', and it is common practice to insinuate that researchers and observers critical of the science on second-hand smoke have financial ties with the tobacco industry.

As Mair and Kierans (2007) have highlighted, tobacco research is increasingly defined by a commitment to the goals of tobacco control. 'Legitimate' tobacco research explicitly aims to reduce the burden of tobacco-related disease and is defined in contrast to industry research aimed at promoting tobacco use. In this moralized framing there can be no interested observers. As befits a substance in the new public health's 'Axis of Evil', the mainstream view appears to be that 'if you're not with us, you're against us'. This growing polarity in tobacco scholarship is, in some ways, comparable to that which Gard (this volume) describes in the field of obesity research, which is organized around the opposition between two broad camps: 'obesity alarmists' and 'obesity sceptics'. However, the polarity is even more pronounced in the case of tobacco research insofar as *any* research critical of tobacco-control policies is often dismissed by public-health officials and non-smokers' rights groups[1] as parroting the views of the tobacco industry.[2]

In this chapter I do not intend to draw any conclusions about the 'truth' regarding second-hand smoke. Rather, I am interested in examining this issue as a discursive formation (Foucault 1970): in particular, *why* second-hand smoke, also known as 'environmental tobacco smoke', 'passive smoking' and 'involuntary smoking',[3] has become such a central focus in tobacco control and public-health policy. I consider contemporary developments in tobacco-control policy in relation to the available evidence base regarding the health impacts of second-hand smoke and its distinctive symbolic attributes. My key goal is to demonstrate that the subjectively experienced abjectness of cigarette smoke far more than the 'objectively' demonstrable harms to health it causes ultimately explain both popular and public-health responses to the substance.

The rise of second-hand smoke as a public-health issue

While the late-twentieth and early-twenty-first century can be characterized by an extreme preoccupation with second-hand smoke, objections to such smoke are longstanding and first appeared in tandem with the emergence of widespread tobacco use in Europe in the late-sixteenth century. For example, in 1604, King James VI of Scotland wrote an anti-smoking pamphlet, *A Counterblaste to Tobacco*, in which he attacked both tobacco use and second-hand smoke, noting:

> And for the vanities committed in this filthy custom, is it not both great vanity and uncleanness that at the table, a place of respect, of

cleanliness, of modesty men should not be ashamed to sit tossing of tobacco pipes and puffing of the smoke of tobacco one to another making the *filthy smoke and stink thereof to exhale athwart the dishes and infect the air* when very often men that abhor it are at their repast.

(n.p., emphasis added)

Annoyance about exposure to tobacco smoke was also a significant element in the anti-smoking movement of the nineteenth century (Sullum 1998). For example, an image from 1886 titled 'The smoke nuisance' shows a man smoking in a train carriage and subjecting its occupants to copious fumes (see Figure 5.1). A man is depicted opening a window and a little boy cries plaintively, 'Mama! I am so sick.' The mother is holding a handkerchief and says, 'Oh! What a horrible smell!'

Interesting are connections made even in this early period between smoke, sickness and contamination. Such connections were made even more explicitly in 1911 when Charles Pease argued that

The right of each person to breathe and enjoy fresh and pure air – *air uncontaminated by unhealthful or disagreeable odours and fumes* – is a constitutional right, and cannot be taken away by legislatures and courts, much less by individuals pursuing their own thoughtless or selfish indulgence.

(In Sullum 1998: 33, emphasis added)

Although these arguments prefigure contemporary assertions of non-smokers' rights, it was not until the 1970s that the second-hand smoke

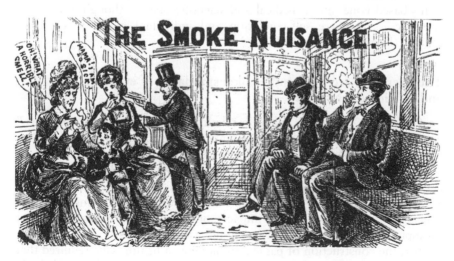

Figure 5.1 1886 engraving on second-hand smoke (image available from National Library of Medicine – no copyright restrictions).

'issue' emerged as a central platform of the anti-tobacco lobby (Sullum 1998; Berridge 1999). However, this shift in focus proved highly successful as it allowed the anti-smoking lobby to further its agenda whilst sidestepping accusations of paternalism (Kagan and Vogel 1993; Bayer and Colgrove 2004). As Kagan and Vogel (1993: 39) note:

> Although the activists' underlying goals may be paternalistic – to induce inconvenienced smokers to quit, to delegitimate smoking and thereby discourage smokers and potential smokers – their arguments could now take a classically libertarian form: 'your freedom to choose to smoke ends where my airspace, and my right to breathe unhazardous air, begins.'

This allowed tobacco-control advocates to push for changes that would have been politically unpalatable if they had been pursued directly (Bayer and Colgrove 2004: 953).

Such efforts to lobby for the regulation of smoking occurred within a context of scientific uncertainty about the nature of the harms of second-hand exposure to tobacco smoke (Zimring 1993; Brandt 1998; Sullum 1998; Berridge 1999; Bayer and Colgrove 2004). Examinations of the historical context of tobacco-control policies in the United Kingdom (Berridge 1999), the USA (Sullum 1998) and Canada (Asbridge 2004) have shown that moves to restrict smoking were based less on scientific research than the issue of non-smokers' rights and the pressure placed on local municipalities by advocacy groups. However, the medical legitimacy provided by research findings about the health impacts of second-hand smoke allowed tobacco-control advocates to redefine passive smoking from a moral and rights-based issue into a medical and scientific one – although 'this was a scientific issue where self-regulation and individual morality were still central' (Berridge 1999: 1192).

The science of second-hand smoke: standards of evidence and public-health action

As Gusfield (1981: 3) has noted in relation to drink-driving: ' "objective" conditions are seldom so compelling and so clear in their form that they spontaneously generate a "true" consciousness.' Similarly, the rise of second-hand smoke as a public-health 'problem' cannot be understood as a natural consequence of the 'objective' dangers it poses (Jackson 1994; Sullum 1998; Berridge 1999). Unlike the research on smoking and lung cancer, studies on the health impacts of second-hand smoke were not prompted by unexplained increases in disease (Gostin 1997; Sullum 1998). Rather, the construction of passive smoking as a health issue required that epidemiology infiltrate the spaces and connections between the visible body of the smoker and the invisible body of the passive smoker (Jackson 1994).

Although these links are understood to have been rendered progressively more visible by technical developments and increasing medical insight, Jackson (1994) convincingly demonstrates the ways these links were actively produced by a particular logic.

Central to the scientific literature on second-hand smoke is a preoccupation with the constituents of the smoke itself: cigarette smoke was quickly reduced to its chemical components (e.g. carbon monoxide, tar, ammonia, benzene, etc.), which were then classified in relation to their likely impact on health (Jackson 1994). However, while medical science could measure the carbon-monoxide concentration of cigarette smoke, it was ill-equipped to conceptualize the risk of exposure to such substances by the disease-free, and therefore *invisible*, passive smoker (Jackson 1994: 434).

As Jackson notes, scientific precision disappears when the actual effects of this smoke are discussed. Thus, a 1986 article by Peto and Doll states: 'it is *generally* accepted that safe thresholds are *unlikely* to exist for most carcinogens ... exposure to ambient smoke must be *assumed* to cause lung cancer in non-smokers' (cited in Jackson 1994: 436, emphasis in original). In light of these intrinsic uncertainties, Jackson points to the critical role played by biomarkers, particularly cotinine, in legitimizing the links between the visible smoker and the invisible passive smoker. Although cotinine is a metabolite of nicotine, which is not in itself carcinogenic, its importance resides in its presumed indexical relationship with other less-visible constituents. 'These remain hidden in the human body and yet can be revealed by way of discursive associations' (Jackson 1994: 439).

Although a considerable amount of research has been conducted into the toxicology of second-hand tobacco smoke since the publication of Jackson's paper, his basic observations remain pertinent. Thus, when considering the mechanisms through which second-hand smoke leads to health impacts, the latest Surgeon General's report notes, 'the mechanisms by which secondhand smoke causes lung cancer are *probably similar* to those observed in smokers' (USDHHS 2006: 46). Yet, despite ongoing uncertainty about the exact mechanisms through which second-hand smoke leads to disease, over the last thirty years the wording of the Surgeon General's reports has become strikingly absolute in tone. For example, the 1972 Surgeon's General's report concluded that: 'the effect of exposure to carbon monoxide may on occasion, depending upon the length of exposure, be sufficient to be harmful to the health of an exposed person' (USDHHS 1972: 7). Contrast this with the wording of the 2006 report, which concludes: 'Exposure of adults to secondhand smoke has *immediate* adverse effects on the cardiovascular system and *causes* coronary heart disease and lung cancer.... The scientific evidence indicates that there is *no risk-free level of exposure* to secondhand smoke' (USDHHS 2006: 9, emphasis added).

So what exactly are the established risks of second-hand smoke exposure? According to the 2006 Surgeon General's report (USDHHS 2006), the pooled evidence indicates a 20-to-30 per cent increase in the risk of lung cancer and a 25-to-30 per cent increase in the risk of coronary heart disease associated with living with a smoker (USDHHS 2006: 15). The relative risk is therefore between 1.20–1.30 in the majority of studies (USDHHS 2006) – a reasonably weak relationship in epidemiological terms.[4] Moreover, as Gostin (1997) points out, the Surgeon General's more recent scientific conclusions regarding the causal link between second-hand smoke and disease lack the rigour of earlier reports, failing to clearly state the conditions required in order for significant health risks to occur. As Gostin asks: 'At what level of exposure does the risk occur? How serious a risk exists compared with other environmental risks, such as automobile emissions? What kinds of involuntary smoking or what settings pose the risks?' (1997: 347).

The conclusions drawn by the Surgeon General also pose a considerable contrast to those regarding other identified health hazards with similarly established levels of risk. For example, over the past twenty years there has been considerable debate in the epidemiological literature about the relationship between alcohol use in women and breast-cancer risk (e.g. Steinberg and Goodwin 1991; Ellison *et al.* 2001; Nagata *et al.* 2007). Early reviews of the alcohol–breast-cancer link were highly equivocal, failing to find support for a clear causal relationship between them based on the low relative risks found and the high percentage of studies that failed to find evidence of a significant effect (e.g. Steinberg and Goodwin 1991).

More recent reviews have been slightly less tentative in their conclusions. Key *et al.* (2006), in a meta-analysis of ninety-eight studies, found an excess risk associated with alcohol drinking of 22 per cent, with each additional 10 grams of ethanol per day associated with a 10 per cent increase in risk. They conclude:

> *Taking account of shortcomings in the study base and methodological concerns*, we confirm the alcohol–breast cancer association. We compared our results to those of an individual patient data analysis, with similar findings. We conclude that the association between alcohol and breast cancer *may* be causal.
>
> (2006: 759, emphasis added)

Boyle and Boffetta take a stronger stance on the causality of the link between alcohol and breast cancer, but still acknowledge the risk to be 'quite small', with a 'gradient of increasing risk of breast cancer associated with increasing levels of alcohol consumption' (2009: S5). Bearing in mind the similar relative cancer risks that alcohol consumption and second-hand smoke exposure entail, and the dose–response relationship evident in each case, the Surgeon General's conclusion that there is 'no risk-free level' of second-hand smoke exposure seems strikingly intemperate in comparison.

The radically different assessment of risk levels that are 'objectively' similar bears out Brandt's (1998) point that thresholds for public regulation and intervention are socio-political phenomena. As he notes:

> They vary not only by the ability of epidemiology to specify a given risk, at a given level, but rather by the cultural process of how a given risk is publicly perceived and understood. Where and how is the risk generated? Are there reasons for tolerating a particular risk, or not? Who is responsible for generating the risk and what is their social status? What are the available mechanisms for regulation and enforcement? Finally, who is at risk? Are they actors in the risk, or are they passive victims? Are they innocent?
>
> (1998: 171)

Thus, while alcohol use and exposure to tobacco smoke may carry similar cancer 'risks', one risk is seen to result from voluntary exposure and the other from involuntary exposure. Most importantly, the 'victims' of second-hand smoke are 'innocents' – adorable infants are a staple of smoke-free campaign imagery (see Figure 5.2).

It was the identification of harms to 'innocent victims', primarily children and women, that cemented the validity of the second-hand smoke issue (Kagan and Vogel 1993; Brandt 1998; Berridge 1999; Bayer and

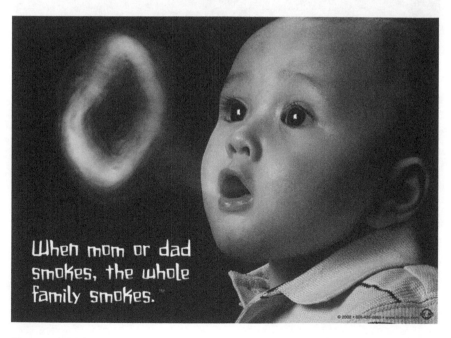

When mom or dad smokes, the whole family smokes.

Figure 5.2 Tobacco-prevention poster depicting passive-smoking infant (reprinted with the permission of State of Health).

Colgrove 2004). As Brandt (1998: 170) asks: 'How persuasive did the data on passive smoking need to be, when the harms that were identified were typically inflicted on "non-consenting" women and children?'

Thus, despite the limitations of the available evidence base beyond the context of intensive, long-term exposure, the position that 'no amount of second-hand smoke is safe' has achieved hegemonic status in the field of

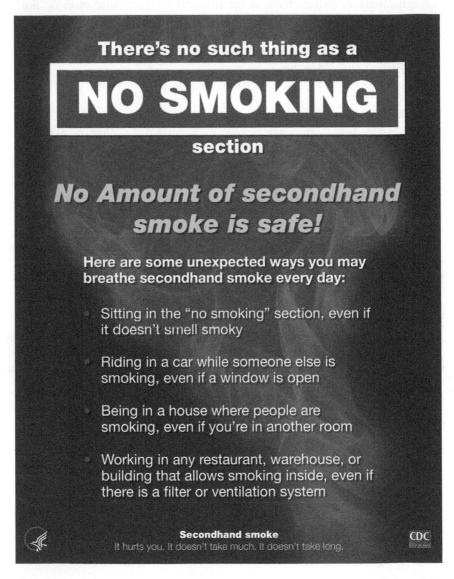

Figure 5.3 CDC second-hand-smoke poster (reprinted with the permission of the CDC).

public health (see USDHHS 2006). For example, a poster from the US Centers for Disease Control and Prevention (CDC) informs the public of the dangers of 'sitting in a "no smoking" section, even if it doesn't smell smoky' and 'being in a house where people are smoking, even if you're in another room' (Figure 5.3). In this framework, all exposures are treated as equivalent: second-hand smoke 'hurts you. It doesn't take much. It doesn't take long.' It is therefore unsurprising that outdoor smoking bans are gaining traction, despite the fact that the established risks associated with such exposure are virtually non-existent (Chapman 2000, 2008).

Invasion and the dissipation of bodily boundaries

Tobacco smoke itself forms a prominent and fetishized visual feature of tobacco-control imagery. The fetishistic nature of second-hand smoke is particularly evident in Figure 5.4, a poster from State of Health, an organization that creates tobacco-prevention and other health-promotion materials aimed primarily at school children. Despite the more lurid B-movie imagery of the poster, the message in both Figure 5.3 and Figure 5.4 is virtually identical: second-hand smoke is an uncontainable, invasive 'killer'.

As Dennis (2006) has previously noted,[5] the frame of invasion is integral to depictions of smoking in tobacco-control campaigns: cigarette smoke refuses to be contained. In anthropological terms, cigarette smoke is a liminal substance (Turner 1967): powerful 'matter out of place' (Douglas 1966 [1996]; see also Manderson 1995). It is precisely these qualities that made tobacco smoke a central component of religious rituals amongst both North and South American Indians, who esteemed it for its sacred, protective and purificatory powers (see Wilbert 1987; Winter 2000). Moreover, as Klein (1993) and Dennis (2006 and this volume) have argued, such transgressive qualities are also intimately connected with the contemporary pleasures of smoking.

Although smoke is intrinsically transitive, a distinctive feature of cigarette smoke is its connection with the human body. Chapman (2000, 2008) has observed the very different reactions cigarette smoke and smoky campfires or barbeques evoke, despite the similar range and volume of carcinogenic particulates and gases both expel. He attributes this to the perceived romance of the smoky campfire in contrast to the perception of second-hand smoke as a 'quintessential imposed risk' linked with the possibility of feared outcomes such as lung cancer (2000: 95). However, in my view the most fundamental difference between assessments of these two types of smoke is that one is connected with organic matter and the other is connected with *the human body*.[6] As Brandt (1998: 168) notes, the term 'second-hand smoke' itself contains the ominous implication that someone else has used it first.

Few scholars have explicitly attempted to theorize these dimensions of cigarette smoke, although notable exceptions include the work of Poland

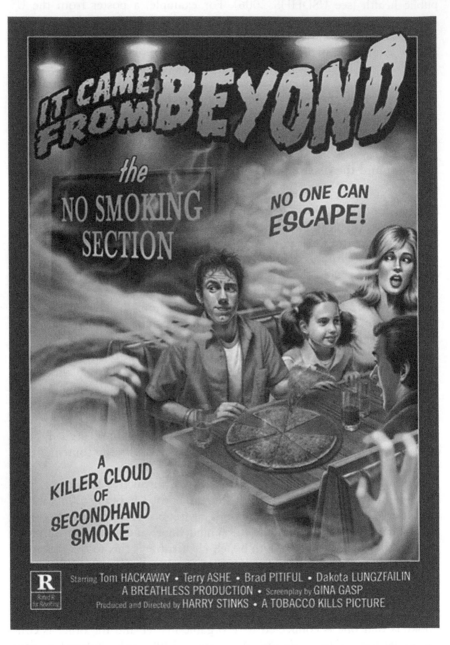

Figure 5.4 Tobacco-prevention poster on second-hand smoke (reprinted with the permission of State of Health).

(2000) and Dennis (2006). Poland (2000) argues that contemporary reactions to second-hand smoke need to be contextualized in relation to the growing importance of etiquette and bodily control to middle-class sensibilities since the eighteenth century. He argues that increasing individualization has heightened awareness of personal space and violations of such space. He writes:

> Environmental tobacco smoke invades the most intimate reaches of the body of physically copresent non-smokers, allowing for the violation of personal space by others at a physical distance in indoor environments. The social class dynamics underlying these 'sensibilities', as well as the social class distribution of smoking, sheds new light on why regulations on smoking have been most swiftly applied to environments with a preponderance of middle and upper classes.
>
> (Poland 2000: 8)

Using a phenomenological lens, Dennis (2006) similarly notes that cigarette smoke makes connections between bodies. While some of these connections may be desirable – such as with the post-coital cigarettes enjoyed by two lovers,[7] other connections may be highly undesirable and unwanted. As Dennis argues, by making connections between bodies, cigarette smoke dissolves the boundaries between them. 'The smoke that goes in is not the same as the smoke that comes out; tasting smoke makes the smoke part of us, and makes us part of smoke' (2006: 48).

Thus, while cigarette smoke crosses boundaries in general, I would argue that it is the dissolution of *bodily boundaries* in particular that make it so uniquely positioned within contemporary public-health discourse. As Mary Douglas has famously noted: 'all margins are dangerous.... Matter issuing from them is marginal stuff of the most obvious kind. Spittle, blood, milk, urine, faeces or tears by simply issuing forth have traversed the boundary of the body' (Douglas 1966 [1996]: 122). So, too, has second-hand smoke. In the language of Julia Kristeva (1982), second-hand smoke is abject: an in-between, ambiguous, composite substance that destroys the boundaries between what is 'me' and what is 'not me'. As Kristeva (1982: 4, emphasis added) writes, 'It is thus *not lack of cleanliness or health* that causes abjection but what disturbs identity, system, order. What does not respect borders, positions.'

The abject nature of cigarette smoke is starkly highlighted in the language of disgust that non-smokers and ex-smokers (and occasionally smokers themselves) use to describe it. For example, Ann, a middle-aged general physician interviewed as part of my research into smokers' and GPs' interactions about smoking,[8] stated in no uncertain terms: 'I think it's *disgusting*. I *hate* the smell of it.' Ex-smokers were often equally damning. Jackie, a woman in her twenties, described her newly acquired repugnance of cigarette smoke using similarly strong words: 'especially after you quit it smells *disgusting*.' As an emotion, disgust tends to embody ideas about contamination (Nussbaum 2004), with its attendant imagery of borders under attack.

As these accounts suggest, central to the abject, contaminating qualities of second-hand smoke is its smell. Although such smoke is also signified visually, its most powerful referent is olfactory: smoke is often smelled long before it is seen and long after the smoke itself (and the cigarette that produced it) has been extinguished. It is smoke's 'tell-tale' trace. Jack, a retired GP, described the ways in which the smell of smoke made it impossible for the smokers amongst his patients to hide their smoking status from him: 'when someone comes in and they smoke, I mean, not only do they look like they smoke but you can smell smoke on them.'

Marks (2002) argues that smell is the most mimetic of the senses: it acts on our bodies before we are conscious of it. Moreover, we cannot actively avoid smells or guard ourselves from the bodily invasion they entail. As Le Guérer (1990: 175) notes:

> The smell that enters the lungs establishes a contact 'even more intimate' than the one between taste and the receptor cavities of mouth and throat. Furthermore, unlike oral absorption, which is a deliberate act, olfactory perception is almost always involuntary. A smell is unavoidable, for it cannot be either voided or avoided through a rejective process like vomiting.

Thus, it is the smell of second-hand smoke as well as the visible signs that accompany it that are integral to present assessments of the health risks it poses.[9] Indeed, it is precisely the mimetic, embodied effects of smoke's odour that appear to be driving recent research into the health impacts of 'third-hand smoke': residual tobacco smoke 'contamination' (see Winickoff *et al.* 2009).

These embodied effects are also central to the ready acceptance of the science of second-hand smoke amongst the public. For example, Malone *et al.* (2000), in their analysis of newspaper coverage of passive smoking, have found that 'evidence' regarding the harmfulness of second-hand smoke tended to appeal to phenomenological arguments over scientific evidence. Thus, smelly clothes and watery eyes were used as experiential evidence to support scientific claims. As the authors note: 'In the end, the science of passive smoking was used to confirm what "everyone" already *knew through everyday experience*, and to establish socially legitimated "facts" that provided official justification for subsequent action' (Malone *et al.* 2000: 719, emphasis added).

I would suggest that the mimetic, affective and abject qualities of second-hand smoke have helped to naturalize and disguise the symbolically constructed nature of the association between smoke and disease, and its 'dangerous' and 'unhealthy' qualities have now become self-evident. This

explains why in the space of less than two decades, social and legal attitudes towards second-hand smoke have been so fundamentally transformed: the powerful mimetic and embodied response second-hand smoke
produces has been successfully harnessed by the anti-tobacco lobby for
instrumental purposes. To paraphrase Marks (2002),[10] in this framework
the experiential aspects of second-hand smoke have been co-opted in
service of a socio-political movement.

Conclusion

Clearly, the science of second-hand smoke cannot be divorced from the cultural context central to its emergence as a public-health issue. Whilst objections to second-hand smoke are longstanding, it is only in the past two
decades that it has been singled out for uniform attack as a dangerous and
polluting substance. On the basis of the comparatively minor established
health risks second-hand smoke exposure poses – risks that are most concrete in the context of long-term and intensive exposure – strikingly absolute
legislation has been enacted to remove all traces of second-hand smoke from
indoor public places and, increasingly, outdoor public spaces as well.

I have tried to demonstrate that public-health responses to second-hand
smoke cannot be divorced from the abject and mimetic effects of this
smoke. Smoke dissipates bodily boundaries and undermines the separation
between self and other in ways highly problematic in the context of late-
industrial capitalist life. Its powerful mimetic effects disguise the highly
artificial medicalized meanings second-hand smoke has come to hold over
the past twenty-five years. Thus, the intrinsic 'risk' it poses, regardless of
intensity of exposure, has become apparently self-evident: a cultural and
medical 'fact' requiring little explication.

Notes

1 Although anti-smoking organizations and public-health agencies are not synonymous, there is a close connection between them. For example, most of the
members of the Framework Convention Alliance (FCA), the organization
responsible for implementing the WHO Framework Convention on Tobacco
Control treaty, are anti-smoking organizations and the head office of FCA is
the US branch of ASH (Action on Smoking and Health) – a strident non-
smokers' rights organization.

2 For example, following the publication of a recent paper of mine critical of
tobacco denormalization policies and their impact on smokers (Bell *et al.* 2010),
the Canadian Non-Smokers Rights Association immediately responded by
calling the research 'shoddy' and accused it of 'parrot[ing] the tobacco industry's attempt to portray anti-smoking efforts as an attack on individuals' (see
Blackwell 2010).

3 As Brandt (1998) has noted, each of these terms has particular social and political implications. For example, 'involuntary' smoking emphasizes the 'voluntary' and intentional nature of smoking, while 'environmental tobacco smoke'
invites public concern about smoking as an environmental hazard. According to

Brandt (1998: 168), 'each of these terms had alternate and reinforcing qualities in spurring this second anti-tobacco revolution'. I have chosen to use the term 'second-hand smoke' because this is the one most commonly used by the public-health agencies I examine in this chapter. As I go on to discuss, this term emphasizes the 'used' nature of this smoke, which I believe is central to its contemporary status as physically and symbolically defiling.

4 It is worth noting that the documented risks of active smoking exponentially outweigh the risks associated with passive smoking (USDHHS 2006). The relative risks associated with long-term, heavy smoking are between 12.7 and 23.3 – an 1,100 to 2,200 per cent increase in risk (ACS 2008). Tobacco-control campaigns on second-hand smoke have worked so well there is some evidence that the public now overestimate the risks of second-hand smoke exposure in relation to active smoking (e.g. Halpern-Felsher and Rubinstein 2005). The iatrogenic consequences (Castel 1991) of such overestimates have been little explored.

5 Dennis (2006) primarily focuses on the frame of internal invasion depicted in tobacco-prevention images of the internal organs of the body being encompassed by tobacco. However, the frame of external invasion is equally integral to tobacco-control campaigns connected with second-hand smoke.

6 Although a distinction is made between mainstream smoke (smoke exhaled by the smoker) and sidestream smoke (smoke directly from the cigarette itself), and sidestream stroke is the more toxic of the two (USDHHS 2006), as the term 'second-hand' smoke itself suggests, it is the smoke exhaled by the smoker that is the primary focus of attention.

7 The desirability of such smoky connections may help to explain the high degree of resistance to smoking bans in bars and nightclubs – venues where connections between bodies are actively sought out.

8 This research examined the impact of social de-normalization strategies on interactions between smokers and GPs about smoking. Twenty-five smokers and ten GPs were interviewed between 2008–2009. The study was funded by the Canadian Institutes of Health Research.

9 Although the abjectness of such smoke was de-emphasized in mainstream discourse on smoking for much of the twentieth century (perhaps because smells, despite their liminal qualities, are habituating), it is certainly present in anti-smoking propaganda throughout history, with its focus on 'filthy' and 'contaminating' fumes.

10 Marks (2002) refers to the commercial applications of smell as a marketing tool, despite its affective and mimetic qualities.

References

ACS (2008) *Smoking and Cancer Mortality Table*, American Cancer Society. Online, available at: www.cancer.org/docroot/PED/content/PED_10_2X_Smoking_and_Cancer_Mortality_Table.asp (accessed 15 June 2009).

The Age (2007) 'Smoking ban for cars in force in SA', *The Age Online*. Online, available at: www.theage.com.au/news/National/Smoking-ban-for-cars-in-force-in-SA/2007/05/31/1180205402770.html (accessed 23 July 2008).

Asbridge, M. (2004) 'Public place restrictions on smoking in Canada: Assessing the role of state, media, science and public health advocacy', *Social Science and Medicine*, 58: 13–24.

Bayer, R. and Colgrove, J. (2004) 'Science, politics, and ideology in the campaign against environmental tobacco smoke', *American Journal of Public Health*, 92(6): 949–954.

Bell, K., Salmon, A., Bowers, M., Bell, J. and McCullough, L. (2010) 'Smoking, stigma and tobacco 'denormalization': Further reflections on the use of stigma as a public health tool', *Social Science and Medicine*, 70: 795–799.

Berridge, V. (1999) 'Passive smoking and its pre-history in Britain: Policy speaks to science?', *Social Science and Medicine*, 49: 1183–1195.

Blackwell, T. (2010) ' "Shaming" smokers makes it harder to quit: Study', *National Post*. Online, available at: www.nationalpost.com/news/canada/story. html?id=2417574 (accessed 4 April 2010).

Bloch, M. and Shopland, D. (2000) 'Outdoor smoking bans: More than meets the eye', *Tobacco Control*, 9: 99.

Borthwick, F. (2000) 'Olfaction and taste: Invasive odours and disappearing objects', *The Australian Journal of Anthropology*, 11: 127–140.

Boyle, P. and Boffetta, P. (2009) 'Alcohol consumption and breast cancer risk', *Breast Cancer Research*, 11 (Suppl. 3): S3–S6.

Brandt, A.M. (1998) 'Blow some my way: Passive smoking, risk and American culture', in S. Lock, L.A. Reynolds and E.M. Tansey (eds) *Ashes to Ashes: The History of Smoking and Health*, Amsterdam: Rodopi, pp. 164–187.

CACBC (2008) *Imagine! Campaign*, Clean Air Coalition of BC. Online, available at: www.cleanaircoalitionbc.com/imagine_campaign.html (accessed 16 June 2009).

Canadian Press (2007) 'MPP bill calls for smoking ban in cars with minors', *CTV. ca*. Online, available at: www.ctv.ca/servlet/ArticleNews/story/ CTVNews/20071206/no_smoking_bill_071206 (accessed 23 July 2008).

Castel, R. (1991) 'From dangerousness to risk', in G. Burchell, C. Gordon and P. Miller (eds) *The Foucault Effect: Studies in Governmentality*, Hemel Hempstead: Harvester Wheatsheaf, pp. 281–298.

Chapman, S. (2000) 'Banning smoking outdoors is seldom ethically justifiable', *Tobacco Control*, 9: 95–97.

Chapman, S. (2008) 'Should smoking in outside public places be banned? No', *British Medical Journal*, 337: a2804.

City of Vancouver (2008) *Health By-Law No. 9535*, Vancouver: City of Vancouver.

City of White Rock (2008) *The Corporation of the City of White Rock Bylaw 1858*, White Rock: City of White Rock.

Dennis, S. (2006) 'Four milligrams of phenomenology: An anthrophenomenological analysis of smoking cigarettes', *Popular Culture Review*, 15(4): 41–57.

Douglas, M. (1966; reprinted 1996) *Purity and Danger: An Analysis of the Concepts of Pollution and Taboo*, London: Routledge.

Ellison, R.C., Zhang, Y., McLennan, C.E. and Rothman, K.J. (2001) 'Exploring the relation of alcohol consumption to risk of breast cancer', *American Journal of Epidemiology*, 154(8): 740–747.

Foucault, M. (1970) *The Order of Things*, New York: Pantheon.

Gostin, L. (1997) 'The legal regulation of smoking (and smokers): Public health or secular morality?', in A.M. Brandt and P. Rozin (eds) *Morality and Health: Interdisciplinary Perspectives*, Routledge: London, pp. 331–358.

Le Guérer, A. (1990) *Scent: The Essential and Mysterious Powers of Smell*, New York: Kodansha International.

Gusfield, J.R. (1981) *The Culture of Public Problems: Drink-Driving and the Symbolic Order*, Chicago: University of Chicago Press.

Halpern-Felsher, B.L. and Rubinstein, M.L. (2005) 'Clear the air: Adolescents' perceptions of the risks associated with secondhand smoke', *Preventive Medicine*, 41: 16–22.

Jackson, P.W. (1994) 'Passive smoking and ill health: Practice and process in the production of medical knowledge', *Sociology of Health and Illness*, 16(4): 423–447.

James IV, King (1604) *A Counterblaste to Tobacco*. Online, available at: www.jesus-is-lord.com/kjcounte.htm (accessed 16 June 2009).

Kagan, R.A. and Vogel, D. (1993) 'The politics of smoking regulation: Canada, France, the United States', in R.L. Rabin and S.D. Sugarman (eds) *Smoking policy: Law, Politics and Culture*, New York: Oxford University Press, pp. 22–48.

Key, J., Hodgson, S., Omar, R.Z., Jensen, T.K., Thompson, S.G., Boobis, A.R., Davies, D.S. and Elliott, P. (2006) 'Meta-analysis of studies of alcohol and breast cancer with consideration of the methodological issues', *Cancer Causes and Control*, 17: 759–770.

Klein, R. (1993) *Cigarettes are Sublime*, Durham: Duke University Press.

Kline, R.L. (2000) 'Smoke knows no boundaries: Legal strategies for environmental tobacco smoke incursions into the home within multi-unit residential dwellings', *Tobacco Control*, 9: 201–205.

Kristeva, J. (1982) *Powers of Horror: An Essay on Abjection*, New York: Columbia University Press.

Mair, M. and Kierans, C. (2007) 'Critical reflections on the field of tobacco research: The role of tobacco control in defining the tobacco research agenda', *Critical Public Health*, 17(2): 103–112.

Malone, R.E., Boyd, E. and Bero, L.A. (2000) 'Science in the news: Journalists' constructions of passive smoking as a social problem', *Social Studies of Science*, 30: 713–735.

Manderson, D. (1995) 'Metamorphoses: Clashing symbols in the social construction of drugs', *Journal of Drug Issues*, 25(4): 799–816.

Marks, L.U. (2002) *Touch: Sensuous Theory and Multisensory Media*, Minneapolis: University of Minnesota Press.

Nagata, C., Mizoue, T., Tanaka, K., Tsuji, I., Wakai, K., Inoue, M. and Tsugane, S. (2007) 'Alcohol drinking and breast cancer risk: An evaluation based on a systematic review of epidemiologic evidence among the Japanese population', *Japanese Journal of Clinical Oncology*, 37(8): 568–574.

Nussbaum, M.C. (2004) *Hiding from Humanity: Disgust, Shame and the Law*, Princeton: Princeton University Press.

Poland, B. (2000) 'The "considerate" smoker in public space: The micro-politics and political economy of "doing the right thing" ', *Health and Place*, 6: 1–14.

Repace, J. (2000) 'Banning outdoor smoking is scientifically justifiable', *Tobacco Control*, 9: 98.

Steinberg, J. and Goodwin, P.J. (1991) 'Alcohol and breast cancer risk: Putting the current controversy into perspective', *Breast Cancer Research and Treatment*, 19: 221–231.

Sullum, J. (1998) *For Your Own Good: The Anti-Smoking Crusade and the Tyranny of Public Health*, New York: Free Press.

Thomson, G., Wilson, N., Edwards, R. and Woodward, A. (2008) 'Should smoking in outside public places be banned? Yes', *British Medical Journal*, 337: a2806.

Turner, V. (1967) *The Forest of Symbols: Aspects of Ndembu Ritual*, Ithaca: Cornell University Press.

USDHHS (1972) *The Health Consequences of Smoking*, Maryland: Department of Health and Human Services.

USDHHS (2006) *The Health Consequences of Involuntary Exposure to Tobacco Smoke: A Report of the Surgeon General*, Maryland,: Department of Health and Human Services.

Vergakis, B. (2006) Ban smoking in cars with kids? *Trib.com*. Online, available at: www.casperstartribune.net/articles/2006/04/22/news/regional/f9ff282f05d-b18848725715700558e2b.txt (accessed 23 July 2008).

Walsh, R.A., Paul, C.L., Tzelepis, F., Stojanovski, E. and Tang, A. (2008) 'Is government action out-of-step with public opinion on tobacco control? Results of a New South Wales population survey', *Australian and New Zealand Journal of Public Health*, 32(5): 482–488.

Wilbert, J. (1987) *Tobacco and Shamanism in South America*, New Haven: Yale University Press.

Winickoff, J.P., Friebely, J., Tanski, S.E., Sherrod, C., Matt, G.E., Hovell, M.F. and McMillen, R.C. (2009) 'Beliefs about the health effects of "thirdhand" smoke and home smoking bans', *Pediatrics*, 123: e74–e79.

Winter, J.C. (ed.) (2000) *Tobacco Use by Native North Americans: Sacred Tobacco, Silent Killer*, Oklahoma: University of Oklahoma Press.

Zimring, F.E. (1993) 'Comparing cigarette policy and illicit drug and alcohol control', in R.L. Rabin and S.D. Sugarman (eds) *Smoking policy: Law, Politics and Culture*, New York: Oxford University Press, pp. 95–109.

Part II

Rationality and the ambivalent place of pleasure

6 Permissible pleasures and alcohol consumption

Robin Bunton

Introduction

In 2009 a British newspaper carried an article titled 'A degree of excess for Cambridge's blotto brainboxes', which expressed abhorrence at the spectacle of the country's young intellectual elite stooping to a familiar pattern of 'binge-drinking.' The historic May Ball was described vividly in a style that moral entrepreneurs do so well:

> Some finished face down in the grass by the side of a road. Others had to be taken to hospital with alcohol-influenced injuries. Several had very public brushes with the law. Some, mostly young female, had to be supported on the arms of their friends. Others simply stumbled and hit the deck, lying silently in oblivion.
>
> This was how Cambridge University students celebrated the end of their exams – on a 24-hour drinking, staggering and vomiting marathon that demonstrated that even the brilliant can be brainless. So even though these academically talented young men and women may one day enjoy life's glittering prizes, the early hours of yesterday left Cambridge looking like any other city plagued by mindless yobs and drunks in 21st-century Britain.
>
> (Harris 2009)

The rhetorical strength of this article stems from the perceived threat this style of intoxication poses to sacred academic institutions, as 'Pools of vomit and trails of urine stained ancient walkways and corners of celebrated buildings'.

This story joins many similar newspaper attacks on Britain's so-called binge-drinking culture appearing over the last five years or so and, as such, is perhaps unremarkable. The article does, however, articulate some quite significant features of early-twenty-first-century problems with drug and alcohol pleasures, and highlights the apparent threat 'binging' poses to one iconic centre of reason. Whilst this 'binge culture' had pervaded most city centres in the UK since the late 1990s, in 2009 it was still newsworthy to report on its incursion into the rather more sacrosanct territory of Cambridge and the intellectual elite, particularly when women's drinking was implicated. This article seems an appropriate point of departure when considering the ways in which Western societies evaluate drinking pleasures and the problems it causes for them.

The ways in which a society organizes pleasure, leisure and play tells us much about its core values. This organization varies enormously across time and space, nowhere more than in relation to the pleasures in using drugs and alcohol. In contemporary Western healthcare systems, the governance of drinking and recreational drug pleasures increasingly rely upon dispersed mechanisms of risk-assessment and 'self-management'. Preventive public-health measures are coordinated across a wide variety of public and private bodies. Individuals and communities are encouraged to become conspicuously active citizens.

The merging of moral management and personal health is nothing new. Foucault (1990, 1993) documented similar invocations to 'care of the self' in antiquity. In the context of industrial societies, self-care draws upon expert knowledge and discourses to regulate or govern the quality of life of populations, its health and security in a manner that Rose (1999) refers to as the 'politics of conduct'. By this he refers to the means of governance that extend beyond the formal institutions of the state and focus upon human capacities and behaviours. Regulation of drinking pleasures and problems, for example, is not restricted to the activities of small groups of professionals but is part of a generalized political technology or 'biopolitics' (Hewitt 1991). It is from this point of view that I examine some features of the governance of drinking pleasures and in particular how some pleasures are deemed more or less permissible whilst others are seen as transgressive. I sketch the range of possible drinking and drug pleasures before considering the case of Puritan pleasures, which illustrates the ways in which certain pleasures can be established as permissible and others troubling. Similar techniques of distinction are used, I argue, in recent treatments of the relatively new category of 'binge-drinking' in the UK. The chapter then reflects on ambivalence and contradiction in contemporary consumer capitalism towards the intoxicated body.

The social organization of pleasure

Whilst the study of drug misuse does not exactly ignore pleasure, it has until quite recently afforded it only marginal interest. In part, this may be because non-problematic drug use has been relatively neglected when compared to problematic drug use (Gamble and George 1997; Southgate and Hopwood 2001). With notable exceptions (see, for example, Hinchliff 2001; Measham 2004b; Holt and Treloar 2008), it is difficult to find literature that speaks directly of the pleasures that result from use. Domain assumptions in the drug-problem field direct our attention to the risks to mind, body and society, a bias that has not been apparent in anthropology or in neurological research. There is a history of anthropological study focusing on the non-problematic, everyday use of drugs highlighting cultural/functional benefits (Agar 1985). This approach has sometimes been accused of perpetuating a type of 'problem deflation' (Room 1983), in contrast to a profoundly biomedical perspective in the study of drug use, often reflecting research and service funding (Gefou-Madianou 1992). Neurophysiological work also continues to explore aspects of the positive evaluation of drug pleasures (Gardner and David 1999; Self 2004), as does some of the recent work on well-being and happiness (Layard 2005).

The relative neglect of pleasure in drug and alcohol research is part of a broader difficulty public-health research has with pleasure (Coveney and Bunton 2003; Bunton and Coveney 2010). This neglect matches an even broader neglect of the study of pleasure in Western thought dating back at least as far as Plato, and a privileging of thought over emotions (Gosling and Taylor 1982). Although human happiness was a feature of Enlightenment discourse on politics, treatments of pleasure tended to be rather sanitized (Porter and Mulvey-Roberts 1996). Physical pleasure appears to be particularly troubling to reasoned discourse in the West, and often serves as a critical foil. The more embodied focus in the work of Nietzsche (1966) and Bataille (1987), for example, has provided some twentieth-century feminist writers with a critical vantage point from which to disrupt 'male-stream' assumptions in philosophy (Grosz 1994). In a similar vein, consideration of the types of embodied pleasure can give us critical perspectives on the changing evaluation of pleasure and also, to use Foucault's (1990) term, 'the uses of pleasure'. Previously, John Coveney and I sketched a tentative and far from exhaustive taxonomy of pleasures pertinent to public health (Coveney and Bunton 2003; Bunton and Coveney 2010). We termed these as: disciplined, ascetic, carnal and ecstatic pleasures. We argued that different social and historical circumstances, different systems of thought and expressivity, privilege certain forms of pleasure over others. In this chapter I want to build upon these categories to analyse drinking pleasures and, distinguishing the first two pleasures from the latter, argue that some pleasures are more permissible than others in modern and pre-modern societies. First, I must briefly mention the types of pleasure and in particular the difference between concepts of pleasures that focus on regulation as opposed to the more expressive pleasures.

Disciplined and ascetic pleasures

Certain pleasures appear to derive from the regulation of the body and internal states. *Disciplined* and *ascetic* pleasures are pleasures that have been rationalized or regulated and made safe by reasoned judgement. They contrast to those seemingly vulgar or emotional displays that may be experienced as 'unpredictable', 'perverse' or 'risky'. *Disciplined* pleasure gained ascendency in late-medieval Europe alongside challenges to the ideology of the Catholic Church. During this period, communion with God became more personal and involved reading or listening to the Scriptures with a calm, self-directed attitude. This replaced the communal ritual that characterized the Catholic mass, and public emotional display became subordinated to more cognitive practices for worship as 'innerliness' became sacred, encapsulated in the practice of confession (Foucault 1988). Under the Reformation, pleasure moved away from carnal gratification towards a more sublime state. A range of aesthetic, so-called 'cultivated and civilized', practices emerged (Elias 1982). Similar tendencies can be found in the guidance on appropriate alcoholic drinking that appeared in the nineteenth and early-twentieth centuries as 'drinking sciences' allied themselves with the Church in the name of 'temperance'. Calls for moderate or temperate drinking were directed at the newly urbanized working classes (Harrison 1971; Alasuutari 1992). The moral crusade of the 'temperance' movement of the turn of the twentieth century, by 'othering' certain pleasures as diseases of the will, reinforced a disciplined rational form of drinking pleasure that was moderate and temperate, and placed value on inner-directed self-discipline. *Disciplined pleasure* is arguably at the foundation of many public-health initiatives. Moderation, restraint and tempered practices are integrated into the very fabric of public-health discourse (see also Coveney, this volume). Immediate gratification is relinquished for the pleasure and satisfaction of reasoned self-control.

In contrast to intellectual, cognitive *disciplined* pleasure, *ascetic* pleasure requires the practice of *askesis*, or self-discipline. Practices that managed pleasure by self-control and moderation were apparent in Ancient Greece and can be traced through to early Christian doctrines of virtuous pleasure, asceticism and abstinence, often involving severe fasting and other ascetic rituals. Such ritual denials were an attempt to purify the body, as arousal of bodily passion was considered a contaminant to the soul and a source of sin. Vestiges of such invocations to self-regulation can be seen in contemporary public health's construction of a certain type of self-regulating, healthy citizenship, encapsulated in the incitement to drink within the recommended units of alcohol, for example, or to eat five pieces of fruit and vegetables a day. Popular culture's endorsement of such forms of civility underlie the public outrage and occasioned moral panic when transgression occurs, as in the newspaper article quoted in the opening section of this chapter.

Carnal and ecstatic pleasures

Disciplined and ascetic pleasures introduce enjoyment into regulation in the name of moderation. Ascetic pleasure derives from the control of the body's natural urges – a type of conquering of the body. Both disciplined and ascetic pleasures blend well with Protestant religious ideologies and also those of thrift, diligence and discipline cherished in the development of the early 'spirit of capitalism' (Weber 2002). By contrast, our latter two forms of pleasure – *carnal* and *ecstatic* pleasure – are more suited to the 'consumer capitalism' of the late-twentieth century by virtue of their celebration of the natural body. Carnal and ecstatic pleasures are sensuous, and come from our physical selves and our senses. They are considered to be unanticipated, rather like libidinal urges. These pleasures may be seen as more instinctual and less culturally mediated. Although they can be evoked or assisted by drugs or other means, it is their unanticipated arousal that makes carnal pleasures socially problematic.

Carnal, physical pleasures are simultaneously of the body and of the world, and their expression frequently speaks of a community's shared values. Ritual drug use and drinking practices, for example, frequently co-produce community and establish boundaries of inclusion and exclusion (Becker 1963; Douglas 1966; Gefou-Medaniou 1992; Grund 1993). Indeed, drinking is a common feature of Christian sacred rituals and practices of congregation. The celebration of embodied desire is central to Eucharist and the carnival, for example.

Carnal pleasures seem to have presented the greatest threat to public health. Bodily pleasures associated with 'risky' drug use, like other public-health pollutants, are often portrayed as dangerous, volatile and disordered, and in need of sanitary measures (Armstrong 1983; Crawford 1999, 2000). Similar censure can be found in relation to ecstatic pleasures. Ecstatic pleasures can be found in many spiritual-bonding rituals associated with exotic tribal societies, but there are homologies with more contemporary youthful 'club-culture' and the drug 'Ecstasy'. The rise of such mass use in the 1990s led to discussion of a changing 'post-modern' 'pick and mix' pattern of drug use and drug-use identity that involved a normalization of illicit drugs (Parker and Measham 1994; Shiner and Newburn 1997, 1999; South 1999). Such drug use has mimicked broader shifts in the consumption of goods and services under the influence of consumer culture, which has had a tendency to aestheticize the body and privilege sensory existence in ways reminiscent of the 'carnival' (Featherstone 2007). The increased popularity of intoxicating commodities can be seen as an element of a recent 're-consecration' of existence through the development of 'tribalistic', ritualistic and sensual solidarity (Maffessoli 1996; Mellor and Shilling 1997). The intense pleasurable intoxication experiences of contemporary dance and club cultures seem to offer opportunities for new forms of associations, facilitated by the use of a range of technologies including: lighting, sound, space, drug use and crowds. These newer spaces for such pleasures, however, are socially troubling and often the focus of policy-control and crackdowns such as those experienced in the late-1990s aimed at the 'club scene' (Shapiro 1999). It is the a-social aspect of carnal and ecstatic pleasures that may be troubling.

Drawing on the ideas of Žižek, Bjerg (2008) has argued that certain drugs are more likely to circumvent social and symbolic processes by mainlining to the brain's pleasure centres through the 'pleasure hormone' dopamine (Goldstein 1997). Bjerg argues that, unlike alcohol or cannabis, heroin and cocaine, for example, might pass our sensory system and in this sense affect a 'purely autistic' high or 'jouissance' (as Žižek 1989 would call it), making this drug experience distinct from other forms of consumption. This probably overstates the case for 'pure' states of enjoyment, as even the most intoxicated lifestyles are mediated by some social processes. As an ideal type, however, this approach offers a useful way of theorizing society's preference for some drug pleasures over others, and perhaps also a recurrent ambivalence. Certain drugs may be more carnally potent and therefore beyond social control, making them more threatening to our civil sensibilities. Some of this ambivalence can be attributed to the fact that the drugs market seems to evade government control. A deeper ambivalence, however, stems from a contradiction between the values of production and consumption. Shifts in capitalist social organization based around production value towards those that facilitate consumption have their counterpart in bodily experience. A contemporary ambivalence has been characterized by Mellor and Shilling (1997) as 'the modern baroque body' in which ascetic and aesthetic bodily sensory existence co-exist in tension. This ambivalent sensory economy produces opposing values of production and consumption within public health and health promotion, which results in only ritualistic responses as citizens vainly attempt to become both greater producers and consumers (Crawford 2000). I turn now to consider examples of the ways that pleasures can be both permissible and troubling.

Permissible pleasures

Religious belief is often seen as the source of restraint on pleasure, and most religions contain doctrines that call for restraint if not abstention from various pleasures, particularly those that excite our physical selves. Indeed, some fundamentalist religious groups have come to symbolize asceticism in the extreme, and yet a closer reading of the texts and examination of the lives of such groups reveals a more open and more complex attitude towards pleasure. Invariably there is some space for pleasure and even some invocation to enjoy everyday pleasures as part of a full religious and moral life. For example, Hawthorn's portrayal of New England Puritans in *The Scarlet Letter* left a lasting impression of a joyless, guilt-ridden, hypocritical sect that has only relatively recently been questioned (Miller 1939; Butt 1986; Daniels 1995). Mencken's often-quoted definition of Puritanism as 'The haunting fear that someone, somewhere, may be happy' may have more to do with the promotion of US free-market liberalism than the reality of Puritan lives. The image of the Puritan as a failed ascetic with a dark and brooding psyche has been recast as a much happier, sociable enjoyer of the moderate pleasures of drinking, dancing, sex, sport and socializing (Daniels 1995). The Puritan minister Joshua Moody encouraged the pursuit of moderate pleasures: 'God has given us temporals to enjoy, we should therefore suck the sweet of them, and so do slake our thirst with them, as not to be insatiably craving after more' (Daniels 1995: 7). Puritanism was not simply the wellspring of restriction underlying US liberalism. Rather, it highlights certain contradictions in attitudes towards pleasure:

> A series of conflicting impulses underlay much of this ambivalence: Puritans believed in conformity to doctrine but also in liberty of conscience; they worked for material prosperity but wanted to avoid worldly temptations; they prized social communalism but asserted economic individualism. Each of these pairs (among others) provided alternatives that competed for loyalty both within society as a whole and within the hearts and minds of individuals.
>
> (Daniels 1995: 16)

Perhaps because of these contradictions, incitements to pleasure always also cautioned against ungodly, unlawful, unreasonable and unproductive activities. Drinking and enjoyment were encouraged as long as they did not wander into drunkenness, gluttony or debauchery.

An aptly named eighteenth-century Puritan text, Coleman's *Government and Improvement of Mirth, According to the Laws of Christianity in Three Sermons*, extols the virtues of 'sober' as opposed to other less-moderate types of mirth. This text privileges moderation and calm rationality, and regrets that mirth has a general tendency to degenerate into sin. Mirth, though charming and graceful when it is innocent, could also lead to transgression. It was necessary, therefore, to distinguish between 'virtuous mirth', 'profitable mirth' and 'carnal' and 'vicious mirth'.

> [Once a] licentious manner of expressing our mirth takes over, all possibilities of innocence, neighborly love, or sobriety vanish. The pretence of restraint may be outwardly maintained but disdain is sneered from the eye and contempt is in the smile; tho indeed envy and spite are under the paint; the look is pleasing enough and gay but tis only disguise, a forced laugh while a man's galled and mad at the heart ... a wretch cannot be overjoyed to see a friend but he must curse him and every cup of drink he gets he damns himself.... [T]he wanton man's mirth is ridiculous. He lays aside the man and the gravity of reason and acts the part of a frolic colt. He roars and frisks and leaps.
>
> (Coleman, quoted in Daniels 1995: 18)

Other documents penned by Coleman, such as *A Serious Address to those who Unnecessarily Frequent the Tavern*, argue that recreation and leisure, though Godly, should be governed by reason and virtue. Importantly, these pleasures should not become an end in themselves, as this was to lead to undesirable mirth which might corrupt the Puritan mind. Pleasure was condoned when it enhanced other valued activities such as civic socializing, group recreation or celebration, but when pursued for its own sake, it was ethically troubling.

By constructing boundaries between virtuous and non-virtuous pleasures in this way, Puritan communities attempted to balance and organize the amounts and types of pleasure experienced. Similar acts of distinction can be found with reference to drug pleasures in post-reformation Europe, ostensibly with more secular commitments. The take up of coffee, tea and chocolate in the West in the (late-)seventeenth, eighteenth and nineteenth centuries is illustrative of the development of a taste for more moderate drug pleasures, matched by the increased value placed upon higher consciousness and the mind by emerging merchant and middle-classes. The values of thrift and enterprise increasingly conflicted with intoxication and drunkenness. Although not without controversy, the arrival of coffee was to have a significant impact socially and was welcomed by the late-seventeenth-century middle-classes as a great 'soberer'. The coffee drinker's good sense and business efficiency were seen as evidence of a 'civilizing' effect. Schivelbusch quotes James Howell's text from 1660:

> Tis found already that this coffee drink hath caused a greater sobriety among the Nations. Whereas formerly Apprentices and clerks with others, used to take their morning's draught of Ale, Beer or Wine, which by the dizziness they Cause in the Brain, made many unfit for business, they use now to play the Good-fellows in this wakeful and civil drink.
>
> (1993: 22)

The ideological effect of coffee as a new drug to the West was profound, as was the later impact of tea. Both beverages pharmacologically embodied the values of the Protestant ethic and materially imposed principles of rationality which served to support emerging industrial capitalism. The new drugs literally embodied 'sobriety' and 'temperance', matched bourgeois values and helped redefine drug pleasures in a contra-direction to intoxication. Although the social organization of eighteenth- and nineteenth-century Europe was far from that of Puritan New England, and its scientific orientation towards drug pleasures was distinct, there does appear to be continuities in their approaches to the governance of pleasure – continuities that are apparent in early-twenty-first-century approaches to drug pleasures.

Troubling pleasures

In the last decade, 'binge-drinking' seems to be have become Britain's foremost moral panic, along with concern over rising consumption rates compared to the rest of Europe. Particular concern has been directed at young people and the social and cultural effects that 'Binge Britain' is having on city centres, described by some as 'no-go zones' (Plant and Plant 2006). Local government has reported increases in alcohol-related public-order problems (Home Office 2001: 1), and police data have identified violence 'hot spots' concentrated around town centre licensed premises (Bromley and Nelson 2002; Hughes *et al.* 2008). The origin of this drinking pattern relates directly to the British Labour Party's policy which since 1997 had been aimed at developing the tourist, retail, hospitality and leisure industries by deregulating and relaxing local alcohol trading hours – often in the name of 'Europeanization' and urban regeneration (DCMS 2004: 4). As a result, highly concentrated numbers of young alcohol consumers congregate in city-centre drinking environments which, along with a marketing of the young person's drinking environment, has radically changed the pub and wine bar culture (Hadfield 2006; Hobbs *et al.* 2000, 2003; Measham 2004b; Plant and Plant 2006). The outcome has been that, as Haywood and Hobbs have observed, the contemporary market 'has transformed our town centres into liminal spaces in which individuals are encouraged to play with the parameters of excitement and excess' (2007: 438). This cultural shift fits a longer trend and a shift in alcohol consumption patterns that mimic the hedonistic cultures of the dance drugs scene of the 1980s and 1990s and normalization of sessional drinking to get drunk and experiment with intoxication (O'Malley and Valverde 2004; Measham and Brain 2005). Both pubs and drinks have been tailored to appeal to a new generation of psychoactive consumers, and a distinct drinking pleasure is being promoted and consumed.

The arrival (or, probably more accurately, the re-emergence) of these new preferred styles of drinking have framed drinking pleasure more in the cast of carnal or ecstatic pleasures, in contrast to the prevalence of more moderate pleasures familiar to previous generations. The fact that this is a mass phenomenon, not restricted to particular classes or groups (although the gender equality in this pattern has not gone without comment), has caused a particular problem for government, social-welfare agencies and drug researchers, and a solution or new approach to this drinking pattern has been necessary. As Hayward and Hobbs state:

> Rather than reject a major facet of their own economic policies, and acknowledge the NTE [night time economy] as a criminogenic zone that was negatively impacting upon their own crime and social order targets, the Labour Party instead constructed official discourses that zoned in on the problematic consumer.... Enter the tired and emotional figure of the so-called 'binge' drinker.
>
> (2007: 440)

Binging seems to have become a quasi-scientific category in the UK context even though its nature is far from clear. Berridge (2005) notes that binge-drinking used to refer to the styles of down-and-out drinkers, but this concept has been applied more broadly, in part as a result of its rediscovery by public health epidemiologists in Eastern Europe (McKee *et al.* 2001). This switch has modified approaches to population health. Binge-style drinking has high public visibility and tends to encourage a distinction between 'them' (young people who drink too much and are 'high risk') and 'us' (who may also drink but whose drinking is 'moderate'). In the same report on the lessons to be learned from temperance, Berridge identifies the need for greater clarity on what constitutes binge-drinking and its opposite – moderate drinking – and the ways that such categories divide target groups: a classic public-health partitioning method that constructs the category of the 'other'. This strategy for moderating drinking is strikingly similar to that of the Puritans. By developing boundaries between bodies or groups within the population, we are able to define potentially at-risk, 'polluting' elements for regulation and restraint. 'Better scientific messages' have been called for, as well as better public communication of these messages and more clarity in presenting the options of moderation or abstinence to redress heavy drinking cultures.

Whilst this seems an eminently valid strategy to reduce drinking, the social creation of scientific categories is apparent. From a health-governance perspective, if we are to turn this new breed of drinking hedonists into sensible drinkers and health-risk-managing citizens, then we need to create a new category of behaviour that can be corrected. In doing so, we ignore the market creation of this new type of drinking pattern and redistribute risk from macro policy to individual acts of restraint (see also Room, this volume, for similar points). This individualizing of risk has become a general feature of risk management in health and other areas (Castel 1991). The process also gives some insights into the ways that crisis in the economic realm can be transferred to the cultural realm, as Habermas (1975) has observed more generally.

The redistribution of risk responsibility achieved by this re-classification does not simply shift responsibility towards the healthy citizen; it also calls for action from dispersed organizations including local police and probation services, to local authorities, licensing agencies, and researchers and research organizations. In the UK, for example, the issue has been taken up by the charitable research organization the Joseph Rowntree Foundation, which has commissioned a series of research papers addressing this new social drinking issue (Berridge 2005; Thom and Bayley 2007; Stead *et al.* 2009). The JRF, with roots in the Quaker movement and with a strong reformist and social Fabian influence, has thus become drawn into the coordinated governance of drinking pleasures.

Conclusion

When considering the social organization of drinking pleasures, we can observe particular economies that privilege some forms of pleasure over others. Certain pleasures are singled out for special attention and restraint or exclusion, whilst others are encouraged and facilitated. The fact that pleasures, desires and sensibilities are socially ordered in this way allows us to ask what types of pleasure a society wants. This is rather like Turner's (1992) question, 'What type of bodies does society want?' The answer to this question is revealing in terms of the core social values it expresses.

Here I have tried to highlight some of the ambivalence currently evident in relation to drinking pleasures and the pleasures of 'binge-drinking'. The construction of this category reveals much about the ways that pleasure is currently governed in the name of public health in contemporary consumer capitalism. I have argued that pleasures that are seated more in the physical body than in its social and cultural counterpart (those that John Coveney and I have previously called 'carnal' and 'ecstatic' pleasures) are particularly problematic for the governance of drinking pleasure. By contrast, the pleasures that are taken in the mastery of the physical body ("disciplinary' and 'ascetic' pleasures) are more compatible with the promotion of the moderate or permissible pleasures, and have more appeal for those wishing to govern the drinking habits of individuals. Demarcating the boundary between different types of pleasure may be seen as a useful strategy of governance of the body's pleasures in modern societies. Strategies for identifying and governing 'virtuous pleasures' in Puritan New England bear striking similarities in this respect to contemporary public-health risk-management strategies. Both encourage individual restraint and self-regulation, as well as organizational governance. Both societies display ambivalence towards pleasure in general and drinking in particular, though for quite different reasons. Detailed study of why this is the case, I would argue, is an important area for public-health research.

References

Agar, M.H. (1985) 'Folks and professionals: Different models for the interpretation of drug use', *International Journal of the Addictions*, 20(1): 173–182.

Alasuutari, P. (1992) *Desire and Craving: A Cultural Theory of Alcoholism*, New York: State University of New York Press.

Armstrong, D. (1983) *Political Anatomy of the Body: Medical Knowledge in Britain in the Twentieth Century*, New York: Cambridge University Press.

Bataille, G. (1987) *Eroticism*, London: Marion Boyars.

Becker, H.S. (1963) *Outsiders: Studies in the Sociology of Deviance*, London: Free Press of Glencoe.

Berridge, V. (2005) *Temperance: Its History and Impact on Current and Future Alcohol Policy*, York: Joseph Rowntree Foundation.

Bjerg, O. (2008) 'Drug addiction and capitalism: Too close to the body', *Body and Society*, 14: 1–22.

Bromley, R. and Nelson, A. (2002) 'Alcohol-related crime and disorder across urban space and time: Evidence from a British city', *Geoforum*, 33(2): 239–254.

Bunton, R. and Coveney, J. (2010) 'Drugs' Pleasures', *Critical Public Health*, in press.

Butt, R. (1986) 'Norman Fiering and the revision of Perry Miller', *Canadian Review of American Studies*, 17: 1–25.

Castel, R. (1991) 'From dangerousness to risk', in G. Burchell, C. Gordon and P. Miller (eds) *The Foucault Effect: Studies in Governmentality*, London: Harvester/Wheatsheaf, pp. 281–298.

Coveney, J. and Bunton, R. (2003) 'In pursuit of the study of pleasure: Implications for health research and practice', *Health*, 7(2): 161–169.

Crawford, R. (1999) 'Transgression for what? A response to Simon Williams', *Health*, 3(4): 650.

Crawford, R. (2000) 'The ritual of health promotion', in M. Calnan, J. Gabe and S.J. Williams (eds) *Health, Medicine and Society: Key Theories, Future Agendas*, London: Routledge, pp. 219–235.

Daniels, B.C. (1995) *Puritans at Play: Leisure and Recreation in Colonial New England*, Basingstoke: Macmillan Press Ltd.

Department Of Culture, Media And Sport (2004) *Guidance to the Licensing Act 2003*, London: DCMS.

Douglas, M. (1966) *Purity and Danger*, London: Routledge.

Elias, N. (1982) *The Civilizing Process (Vol. 2): State Formation and Civilization*, Oxford: Blackwell.

Featherstone, M. (2007) *Consumer Culture and Postmodernism*, London: Sage.

Foucault, M. (1988) 'Technologies of the self', in L.H. Martin, H. Gutman and P.H. Hutton (eds) *Technologies of the Self*, Amherst: University of Massachusetts Press, pp. 16–49.

Foucault, M. (1990) *Care of the Self: History of Sexuality*, vol. 3, Harmondsworth: Penguin.

Foucault, M. (1993) *The Use of Pleasure: The History of Sexuality*, vol. 2, Harmondsworth: Penguin.

Gamble, L. and George, M. (1997) 'Really useful knowledge: The boundaries, customs and folklore governing recreational drug use in a sample of young people', in E.P.A. Cheung and D.A. Riley (eds) *Harm Reduction: A New Direction for Drug Policies and Programs*, Toronto: Toronto University Press, pp. 340–362.

Gardner, E.L. and David, J. (1999) 'The neurobiology of chemical addiction', in J. Elster and O.-J. Skog (eds) *Getting Hooked: Rationality and Addiction*, Cambridge: Cambridge University Press, pp. 93–136.

Gefou-Madianou, D. (1992) *Alcohol, Gender and Culture*, London: Routledge.

Goldstein, A. (1997) 'Neurobiology of heroin addiction and of methadone treatment', *American Association for the Treatment of Opioid Dependence*. Online, available at: www.aatod.org/1998–3.html (accessed 10 April 2009).

Gosling, J. and Taylor, C. (1982) *The Greeks on Pleasure*, Oxford: Clarendon Press.

Grosz, E. (1994) *Volatile Bodies: Toward a Corporeal Feminism*, Bloomington: Indiana University.

Grund, J.-P.C. (1993) *Drug Use as a Social Ritual: Functionality, Symbolism and Determinants of Self-Regulation*, Rotterdam: Instituut voor Verslavingsonderzoek.

Habermas, J. (1975) *Legitimation Crisis*, trans. Thomas McCarthy, Boston: Beacon Press.

Hadfield, P. (2006) *Bar Wars: Contesting the Night in Contemporary British Cities*, Oxford: Oxford University Press.

Harris, P. (2009) 'A degree of excess for Cambridge's blotto brainboxes', *Daily Mail*. Online, available at: www.thefreelibrary.com/A+degree+of+excess+for+Cambridge%27s+blotto+brainboxes-a0201851290 (accessed 20 June 2010).

Harrison, B. (1971) *Drink and the Victorians: The Temperance Question in England 1815– 1872*, Pittsburgh: University of Pittsburgh Press.

Hayward, K. and Hobbs, D. (2007) 'Beyond the binge in "booze Britain": Market-led liminalization and the spectacle of binge drinking', *British Journal of Sociology*, 58(3): 437–456.

Hewitt, M. (1991) 'Bio-politics and social policy', in M. Featherstone, M. Hepworth and B.S. Turner (eds) *The Body Social Process and Cultural Theory*, London: Sage Policy, pp. 225–255.

Hinchliff, S. (2001) 'The meaning of ecstasy use and clubbing to women in the late 1990s', *International Journal of Drug Policy*, 12: 455–468.

Holt, M. and Treloar, C. (2008) 'Editorial: Pleasure and drugs', *International Journal of Drug Policy*, 19: 349–352.

Home Office (2001) *Assessing Local Alcohol-Related Crime: A Demonstration Project in Crime and Disorder Partnerships*, London: Home Office Research, Development and Statistics Directorate.

Hughes, K., Anderson, Z., Morleo, M. and Bellis, M. (2008) 'Alcohol, nightlife and violence: The relative contributions of drinking before and during nights out to negative health and criminal justice outcomes', *Addiction*, 103(1): 60–65.

Layard, R. (2005) *Happiness: Lessons from a New Science*, London: Allen Lane.

McKee, M., Shkolnikov, V. and Leon, D. (2001) 'Alcohol is implicated in fluctuations in cardiovascular disease in Russia since the 1980s', *Annals of Epidemiology*, 11: 1–6.

Maffessoli, M. (1996) *The Time of the Tribes: The Decline of Individualism in Mass Society*, London: Sage.

Measham, F. (2004ba) 'The decline of ecstasy, the rise of "binge" drinking and the persistence of pleasure', *Probation Journal*, 51(4): 309–326.

Measham, F. (2004b) 'Play space: Historical and socio-cultural reflections on drugs, licensed leisure locations, commercialisation and control', *International Journal of Drug Policy*, 15(5–6): 337–345.

Measham, F. and Brain, K. (2005) ' "Binge" drinking, British alcohol policy and the new culture of intoxication', *Crime, Media, Culture*, 1(3): 262–283.

Mellor, P. and Shilling, C. (1997) *Re-Forming the Body: Religion, Community and Modernity*, London: Sage.

Miller, P. (1939) *The New England Mind in the 17th Century*, Cambridge, MA: Harvard University Press.

Nietzsche, F. (1966 [1888]) *The Birth of Tragedy*, trans. W. Kaufman, New York: Vintage.

O'Malley, P. and Valverde, M. (2004) 'Pleasure, freedom and drugs: The uses of "pleasure" in liberal governance of drug and alcohol consumption', *Sociology*, 38(1): 25–42.

Parker, H. and Measham, F. (1994) 'Pick 'n' mix: Changing patterns of illicit drug use amongst 1990s adolescents', *Drug Education, Prevention and Policy*, 1(1): 5–13.

Plant, M. and Plant, M. (2006) *Binge Britain*, Oxford: Oxford University Press.

Porter, R. and Mulvey-Roberts, M. (1996) *Pleasure in the Eighteenth Century*, Basingstoke: Macmillan Press.

Room, R. (1983) 'Alcohol and ethnography: A case of problem deflation?', *Current Anthropology*, 25: 169–191.

Rose, N. (1999) *Powers of Freedom: Reframing Political Thought*, Cambridge: Cambridge University Press.

Schivelbusch, W. (1993) *Tastes of Paradise: A Social History of Spices, Stimulants and Intoxicants*, New York: Vintage Books.

Self, D. (2004) 'Regulation of drug-taking and -seeking behaviors by neuroadaptations in the mesolimbic dopamine system', *Neuropharmacology*, 47: 242–255.

Shapiro, H. (1999) 'Dances with drugs: Pop music, drugs and youth culture', in N. South (ed.) *Drugs: Cultures, Controls and Everyday Life*, London: Sage, pp. 17–35.

Shiner, M. and Newburn, T. (1997) 'Definitely maybe not? The normalisation of recreational drug use amongst young people', *Sociology*, 31(3): 511–529.

Shiner, M. and Newburn, T. (1999) 'Taking tea with Noel: The place and meaning of drug use in everyday life', in N. South (ed.) *Drugs: Cultures, Controls and Everyday Life*, London: Sage, pp. 139–159.

South, N. (ed.) (1999) *Drugs: Cultures, Controls and Everyday Life*, London: Sage.

Southgate, E. and Hopwood, M. (2001) 'The role of folk pharmacology and lay experts in harm reduction: Sydney gay drug using networks', *International Journal of Drug Policy*, 12: 321–335.

Stead, M., Gordon, R., Holme, I., Moodie, C., Hastings, G. and Angus, K. (2009) *Tackling Alcohol Harm: Lessons From Other Fields*, York: Joseph Rowntree Foundation.

Thom, B.M. and Bayley, M. (2007) *A New Approach to Prevent and Reduce Alcohol-Related Harm*, York: Joseph Rowntree Foundation.

Turner, B.S. (1992) *Regulating Bodies: Essays in Medical Sociology*, London: Routledge.

Weber, M. (2002) *The Protestant Ethic and the Spirit of Capitalism*, London: Penguin Books.

Žižek, S. (1989) *The Sublime Object of Ideology*, London: Verso.

7 Intoxication, harm and pleasure

An analysis of the Australian National Alcohol Strategy

Helen Keane

Introduction

The Australian National Alcohol Strategy (Ministerial Council on Drug Strategy 2006a) targets intoxication as one of its four priority areas, with the explicit aim of reducing the level of intoxication among drinkers. While the focus on intoxication as a form of undesirable behaviour can be seen as the continuation of a lengthy history of moral concern about the evils of drunkenness, the alcohol strategy presents the issue in the framework of harm reduction (Room 1998). It states that the strategy development process revealed a 'broad consensus' that 'drinking to intoxication' was the most harmful of alcohol-related behaviours, with a significant negative impact on individual and community safety and well-being (MCDS 2006a: 6). The harms associated with intoxication outlined in the strategy include accidental injuries and fatalities (including drowning and fire fatalities), alcohol overdose, motor-vehicle accidents, violence and crime, verbal abuse, family breakdown, risky behaviours such as unsafe sex, and costs related to amenity issues such as cleaning and insurance pay-outs (MCDS 2006a: 11–12). Given this preponderance of negative consequences and high rates of 'excessive single occasion drinking', to use the strategy's term for binge-drinking, it makes sense for the reduction of intoxication to be identified as a public-health priority.

However, while the construction of intoxication as a negative outcome of unsafe patterns of alcohol consumption is epidemiologically incontrovertible, for many drinkers it would represent a clear example of the determined obtuseness of public health when it addresses the risks and pleasures of everyday life. As recent sociological research has shown, for many drinkers, especially young people, intoxication is not a danger to be avoided, but rather a goal to be achieved. Drinking to get drunk, or 'determined drunkenness' as it has been called, is a routine part of a good night out for a significant proportion of young people (Lindsay 2003; Measham 2004; Measham and Brain 2005). And while drunkenness, at least in public, may attract disapproval and legal sanction, drinking to intoxication is still an expected and accepted aspect of youth leisure. The association of intoxication with fun, freedom and spontaneity has been actively exploited and enhanced by the alcohol industry, but this construction of intoxication as a desirable state cannot be reduced to a marketing ploy. While the meaning of intoxication and the kind of behaviour it produces varies across cultures, the notion of 'time-out' from the norms and demands of daily life is prominent, and for young drinkers often combined with a deliberate embracing of risk and enjoyment of intensity (MacAndrew and Edgerton 1969; Beccaria and Guidoni 2002).

This chapter examines the gap between the public-health conception of intoxication as harm and the experience of bodily pleasure valued by many drinkers. On the one hand it can be argued that the purpose of public health is not to simply describe people's behaviour but to attempt to alter it in order to increase well-being. So, in this sense, the gap between the ideal of safe alcohol consumption and actual drinking behaviour is what makes the enterprise meaningful as a public-health project. However, in the case of intoxication there also appears to be a conceptual disjunction that is liable to be counterproductive to efforts to reduce alcohol-related harm. If health discourse understands intoxication as an expendable harm with no redeeming qualities, it will be unable to recognize its attractions as anything other than evidence of individual or cultural pathology. In part, the public-health understanding of intoxication as outside the parameters of moderate and normal alcohol consumption is produced by a model of drinking that separates it from other forms of recreational psychoactive drug use. While there are clearly significant cultural and legal differences between alcohol and other drugs, for many young people, in particular, alcohol is consumed as a psychoactive drug. For them, intoxication is the point of drinking and cannot be separated from its social functions (Brain *et al.* 2000).

Intoxication as harm and pathology

The National Alcohol Strategy is a key document in the government of alcohol consumption in Australia. Described as 'a plan for action', its aim is 'to prevent and minimise alcohol-related harm to individuals, families and communities in the context of developing safer and healthy drinking cultures in Australia' (MCDS 2006a: 2). To this end, the current strategy has four priority areas: intoxication, public safety and amenity, health impacts, and cultural place and availability.

While the strategy begins with a statement about the popularity of alcohol in Australia – its economic importance and its ubiquitous role in relaxation, social interaction, hospitality and celebration – intoxication is excluded from this functional vision of drinking as a part of national culture. Rather, it appears as one of the dangers of alcohol that is too often tolerated or overlooked. The strategy observes that 'none of the health benefits of alcohol are delivered when it is consumed at levels causing intoxication' while social and physical harms to drinkers and those around them are likely to result (MCDS 2006a: 11). While this may be medically valid, the binary construction of benefits and harms ignores the fact that a behaviour like drinking to intoxication is implicated not only in producing health costs but also in producing the economic benefits mentioned earlier. Moreover, the benefits of relaxation, sociability and celebration are not distinct from intoxication, but co-exist with it.

One of the hallmarks of the alcohol strategy is an explicit focus on Australian drinking culture and the customs, values and norms that surround alcohol consumption. While this cultural perspective is valuable in its recognition of the powerful social, economic and political forces that structure individual drinking and provide the context for its meaning, the strategy's commitment to demarcating intoxication as 'other' to normal drinking produces a peculiarly dichotomized picture of alcohol consumption. On one side are desirable drinking cultures which are characterized by moderate and safe drinking (and presumably by sociability and hospitality), while on the other are what the strategy terms at one point 'drunken cultures rather than drinking cultures' (MCDS 2006a: 4). Drunken cultures are marked by excess, intoxication, health costs and other alcohol-related harms. The aim is to transform the drunken cultures of Australia into civilized drinking cultures. But, to be meaningful, the term 'drinking culture' must surely encompass the range of intermeshed practices and consequences that surround alcohol consumption, from the health-enhancing to the potentially fatal. This is particularly the case in Australia, where drinking forms part of the romantic Australian legend, and heavy drinking (at least among White men) is connected to ideals of egalitarianism, camaraderie and reciprocity (Midford 2005). At a deeper level, as Kapferer (1988: 156) argued in his analysis of the role of drinking in Anzac Day celebrations, alcohol consumption in Australia is a traditional sign and symbol of personal autonomy and individual power.[1] Not only is drink seen as fortifying, strengthening and empowering the drinker, its consumption in large quantities demonstrates a masculine ability to tame the power of drink. In this context, government-sponsored messages to limit drinking to moderate levels are easily dismissed as 'nannyism'.

The construction of intoxication as a harm is equally robust in another key Australian public-health document: the National Health and Medical Research Council's *Australian Alcohol Guidelines* (2001). This document presents safe drinking guidelines in terms of standard drinks per day, for the general population and also for 'special groups' such as people with mental-health problems, women who are pregnant and the elderly. It evaluates drinking patterns in relation to both short-term and long-term harm, with short-term harms being those associated with intoxication. The specific guidelines for young people (up to eighteen years) and young adults (eighteen–twenty-five years) suggest a great deal of risk and harm from drinking, balanced by very little benefit, primarily because of the dangers of intoxication. Young adults are identified as the group at highest risk of alcohol-related injury, including road trauma, violence, sexual coercion, falls, accidental death and suicide. Young people face particular risk of violence, accidents and sexual coercion because of loss of inhibitions and decision-making skills, while also being vulnerable to alcohol overdose (NHMRC 2001: 46–49).

Another group identified in the strategy as suffering from high rates of alcohol-related harm is Aboriginal and Torres Strait Islander peoples. The strategy notes that, while indigenous Australians are less likely to drink than the general population, those that do drink are much more likely to do so at risky levels (MCDS 2006a: 10). In a background paper prepared as part of the National Drug Strategy's complementary action plan for Aboriginal and Torres Strait Islander peoples, the vulnerability of this group to harmful drinking is constructed in terms of history and cultural difference (Ministerial Council on Drug Strategy 2006b). The introduction to the paper stresses the detrimental effect of dispossession on the health of indigenous Australians. Harmful patterns of alcohol and drug use are seen as an effect of suffering as well as a cause of suffering: substance use is interpreted as an attempt by individuals to escape from experiences of grief, trauma, loss, anger, alienation, unemployment and despair (MCDS 2006b: 2). As Maggie Brady (2008) has argued, such narratives of exploitation and victimhood can produce a sense of fatalism about Indigenous drinking because they suggest that harmful consumption patterns cannot be changed and that new styles of drinking cannot be learnt.

The background paper also identifies the specific history of alcohol prohibition as a determining factor in Indigenous drinking patterns. Indigenous people were forbidden to drink until the 1960s, thus a style of communal drinking developed based on the consumption of large quantities of alcohol in short periods of time. The paper notes that drinking allowed people to 'be with family, receive news of other family members, to speak their own language, to sing songs, tell stories' (MCDS 2006b: 2). However, because the paper is focused on the devastating harms of drinking for Indigenous individuals and communities, it confines these social benefits to the past. Thus indigenous drinking is excluded from the positive values of hospitality, sociability and relaxation identified as part of Australian drinking culture by the National Alcohol Strategy.

If we turn to a clinical rather than public-health understanding, intoxication is presented as an individual pathology rather than an epidemiologically determined risk. In the DSM-IV, the American Psychiatric Association's diagnostic manual of mental disorders, alcohol intoxication is presented as a type of alcohol-induced disorder, along with alcohol dependence and alcohol abuse. The diagnostic criteria for alcohol intoxication highlight 'clinically significant maladaptive behavioral or psychological changes' such as inappropriate sexual or aggressive behaviour, mood lability and impaired judgement (APA 2000: 176). This definition constructs intoxication as a pathological condition located in an individual: intoxication produces a 'maladaptive' change in the individual's functioning and their capacities are impaired in a predictable and universal way. The National Alcohol Strategy incorporates this kind of psychopathological understanding of intoxication when it states that 'intoxicated persons cannot function within their normal range of physical/cognitive abilities' (MCDS 2006a: 11). Intoxication here is about an individual loss of function and a decrease in capacities, which produces the individual and social risks emphasized in the harm-reduction perspective.

As with the public-health understanding of intoxication, the model of intoxication as 'maladaptive behavioral or psychological changes' is based on a static and de-contextualized vision of human functioning. It is certainly true that when we are drunk there are many things we cannot do well, or indeed at all. But a phrase such as 'the individual cannot function within their normal range of physical/cognitive abilities' ignores the fact that, from the perspective of the drinker at a social event, drinking reduces some capacities but enhances others which are probably more salient. He may not be able to operate machinery safely but he is able to talk and flirt with strangers, dance with abandon and forget his work worries. Intoxication is experienced as enhancement as well as diminishment.

As I have already suggested, the negative evaluation of intoxication in public-health discourse is different from the DSM-IV model because it is made within the framework of harm reduction in which the explicit stance is one of neutrality towards substance use. However, in relation to illicit drug use, harm reduction and minimization have been criticized for their emphasis on the harms of drug use and a concomitant failure to address the issue of pleasure (Mugford 1993; Duff 2004; Moore 2006). As Duff (2004: 388) argues, pleasure is the reason why the majority of drug users are attracted to drug use and therefore harm minimization will remain indifferent to their concerns until it is able to take pleasure seriously.

The public-health discourse on alcohol is considerably more open to pleasure than that addressing illicit drug use. The particular status of alcohol as a socially valued and economically significant commodity has produced a tradition of paradoxical public-health responses to alcohol consumption (Room 1984; see also Room, this volume). Room (1984: 299) argues that until the 1980s alcohol was regarded as a 'vague embarrassment' in the public-health field because highlighting the significant health costs of drinking and arguing for more stringent controls was too reminiscent of temperance views. Contemporary policies continue to eschew measures such as restrictions on availability and tax increases which have been shown to reduce alcohol-related harm, even though awareness of alcohol as a harmful drug has increased (Room *et al.* 2005; Room 1988).

One way that public-health documents such as the National Alcohol Strategy and the NHMRC alcohol guidelines reconcile their focus on reducing harm with alcohol's special cultural position is through the category of risk. The NHMRC guidelines state that for many people alcohol is part of an enjoyable and healthy lifestyle and that the aim is to provide information to enable Australians to 'enjoy alcohol, if they choose to drink, while minimising harmful consequences' (2001: 3). But despite the rhetorical gesture to enjoyment in the introduction, the guidelines concentrate on harm and risk, with patterns of drinking categorized as low risk, risky or high risk.

The prevalence of risk categories in public-health documents on drinking demands some comment here. In the contemporary landscape of medical culture and health consciousness, risk discourse is so widespread and naturalized that its pertinence 'goes without saying', but it is important to recognize that it leads to a particular figuration of everyday practices. As Mary Douglas (1990) has observed, the contemporary concept of risk has departed from an earlier neutral meaning in which risk described the probability of a loss or a gain. Stripped of its connections with positive outcomes and with the element of chance de-emphasized, '*risk* now means danger, *high risk* means a lot of danger' (1990: 3, emphasis in original). Rather than describing a potential harm, risk has come to designate an actual harm in itself; it has become synonymous with harm. Therefore, describing a pattern of alcohol consumption as 'low risk' still emphasizes harm. It suggests that it would still be best to avoid this behaviour if possible. And while the range of harms that are recognized in the drinking guidelines are broad, including the medical, personal and social, the benefits of drinking are restricted to the physiological and objectively measurable, namely protection against heart disease. Therefore, in relation to possible benefits of drinking for young people, the guidelines have only a negative to report, 'the effect of alcohol in protecting against heart disease has been shown to be relevant only for people over about 40 years. There is no evidence to suggest that it is relevant for younger age groups' (NHMRC 2001: 14).

Because pleasure and enjoyment are not counted as genuine benefits in public-health and medical understandings of intoxication, it is difficult to interpret the deliberate and repeated pursuit of intoxication as anything other than irrational and perverse within this framework. If large numbers of young people are drinking at risky levels in a risky way to achieve an abnormal state of reduced functioning, it must be evidence of some deep-seated problem either within individuals or within youth culture as a whole. The familiar discourses of youth vulnerability and low self-esteem frequently feature in explanatory accounts of youth drinking, despite lack of evidence of a link between levels of self-esteem and alcohol abuse or illicit drug use (Emler 2001: 23).[2] The notion that intoxication is a way of communicating inner pain is vividly expressed in the words of one presenter at a 2004 forum on youth binge-drinking, 'What young people who are deliberately getting drunk are doing is sending out a message to you,

saying, "Give me some attention, I need some help, help me ..."'
(Rowswell, cited in Bennett and Bilardi 2004: 10).

While public-health discourse recognizes moderate and civilized drinking as something that can be enjoyed, it cannot speak of the pleasure of intoxication because of its commitment to its elimination. As O'Malley and Valverde (2004: 39) have argued, 'discourses of pleasure would appear to be used governmentally in a selective and directorial fashion'.

The pleasures of intoxication

Outside the parameters of public health, it is clear that there are a range of different pleasures associated with drinking, from the socially valued to the demonized. Speaking eloquently about one's love for Coonawarra Shiraz is a sign of distinction, looking forward to having a few beers with your mates on Friday night signifies a quintessentially Australian form of mateship, but celebrating the joy of getting deliberately and completely pissed would be taken by many to represent a shift from pleasure to pathological excess. As these examples suggest, the class dimensions of different types of alcoholic beverage, drinking venue and styles of consumption cannot be separated from the production of certain highly visible forms of 'problem drinking'. A historical example is provided by the eighteenth-century 'gin epidemic' in which heavy drinking in the London slums was blamed for infant mortality and rising crime (Warner 1994). As Warner highlights, the downward mobility of gin, from a drink exclusively consumed by the middle- and upper-classes to a cheap lower-class beverage was central to the rousing of public opinion against its effects. In a pattern repeated in more recent drug scares, the most vociferous and moralized criticism was aimed at the drinking of lower-class women in general and mothers in particular (Warner 1994: 498).[3]

John Coveney and Robin Bunton's (2003) recent work on the relationship of public health to pleasure enables an exploration of the varied and differentially valued pleasures of drinking. As they point out, public health has an ambivalent relationship to pleasure. On the one hand it is concerned with the development and promotion of well-being and the good life, and contemporary positive conceptions of health seem to necessarily include a notion of pleasure. But on the other hand, pleasure-seeking activities such as sex, eating, drinking and taking drugs are prime sites for the occurrence of unhealthy risk-taking behaviours and are thus often viewed as threats to well-being (Coveney and Bunton 2003: 166).

The tension surrounding pleasure and its management becomes clearer when different forms of pleasure are distinguished. Coveney and Bunton have developed a four-part typology of pleasure: carnal, disciplined, ascetic and ecstatic, which is set out in detail in Bunton's chapter in this volume. The key distinction relevant to drinking is between carnal and disciplined pleasure. At first glance it appears quite simple to map the distinction between carnal and disciplined pleasure onto norms of drinking. On the one hand we have the spectre of excess and intoxication, as vividly represented by a crowd of rowdy youths emerging from a pub or the carnivalesque displays of 'schoolies week' when Australian school-leavers gather *en masse* at beach resorts to celebrate their graduation. On the other, we have the civilized appreciation of a glass of wine with a well-prepared meal and good conversation which exemplifies the moderate enjoyment of alcohol. As in many other arenas of consumption, what public-health alcohol strategies are aiming to do is transform carnal pleasure into disciplined pleasure.

However, different modes of pleasurable drinking do not necessarily map onto a binary model of carnality versus discipline. Because social divisions such as class, race, ethnicity and gender are potently enacted and expressed through drinking practices, what may appear from the outside to be a unitary drinking culture actually comprises many different styles of consumption. For example, in her study of drinking practices in pubs and clubs in Melbourne, Jo Lindsay (2006) develops a distinction between 'commercial' and 'niche' licensed venues which is closely related to social class and the possession of cultural capital. Niche venues tended to be small and aimed for a 'stylish, artistic or alternative aesthetic' (2006: 40). They attracted a slightly older clientele in small mixed-gender groups and sold more expensive drinks such as imported and boutique beer. Commercial venues were large and noisy, welcoming a diverse but generally younger clientele. These venues encouraged high levels of alcohol consumption through pricing, specials and promotions. Raucous and unrestrained 'drunken comportment' was tolerated, including explicit displays of 'heterosexual interaction' such as 'sexualised dancing' and 'overt sexual approaches' (Lindsay 2006: 47). At one level, the commercial/niche distinction can be linked to carnal as opposed to disciplined pleasure, as obvious drunkenness was rarely evident in the niche bars and displays of heterosexuality were 'subtle'. However, the amount of alcohol consumed by niche-venue patrons was still excessive in public-health terms; indeed, the women in these locations were drinking more on average than women in commercial venues (Lindsay 2006: 49).

While social practices of consumption do not neatly conform to undifferentiated and ideal categories of pleasure, the notion of carnal pleasure is particularly helpful when thinking about intoxication because it highlights an obvious element of young people's drinking which tends not to be explicitly addressed in health discourses. This is the consumption of alcohol as a psychoactive drug. Obviously ethanol *is* a psychoactive drug and is enjoyed for its psychoactive effects, even by those drinkers who sip a moderate glass of wine with dinner. But drinking in order to get drunk, in order to enjoy the intensity and euphoria of intoxication and its ability to alter one's sense of self, is to prioritize these psychoactive effects. It is to consume alcohol as a drug. The heavy weekend sessional drinking which is characteristic of contemporary urban youth culture can be understood as in some ways more like the use of Ecstasy or other party drugs, and less like other forms of more moderate alcohol consumption, whether or not alcohol is actually combined with other drugs. Altered states of consciousness are deliberately pursued within environments in which music, lighting and interior design combine to produce an intense and appealing 'nightlife experience' (Lindsay 2003). In this context, intoxication cannot be separated from the enjoyment of alcohol or its role in social interaction.

Cultural criminologists Fiona Measham and Kevin Brain's (2005) compelling account of young people's drinking and drug use in Britain provides insight into this mode of alcohol consumption. Measham and Brain argue that in Britain over the past decade and a half, a new culture of intoxication has emerged amongst young people which includes increased sessional consumption of alcohol and drunkenness as an accepted, and indeed desirable, state. But they note that these developments cannot be understood in isolation from the increased normalization of illicit drug use and the development of 'new psychoactive consumption styles' which combine alcohol and illicit drugs and are willing to 'experiment with and experience states of altered consciousness as a routine part of leisure "time-out"' (Measham and Brain 2005: 265–266). As they state, 'Alcohol consumption has been integrated into this style so that drink and drug use intertwine and celebrate cultures of hedonistic consumption' (2005: 267).

According to Measham and Brain (2005), the new culture of intoxication was enabled and promoted by a range of social, cultural and economic forces including the rise of dance-party culture in the 1990s and the consequent recommodification of alcoholic beverages into a new range of products, the development of flourishing night-time economies based on the commercial exploitation of pleasure and a general rise in hedonistic consumption. I would add that a new psychoactive consumption style can be seen not only in alcohol and drug consumption but also in trends such as the rise of energy drinks, the use of natural supplements such as ginkgo and guarana, and increasingly widespread use of psychoactive prescription drugs for a range of disorders and problems of living. The practice of enhancing one's existence, happiness and productivity through the use of technology, including pharmacological technologies, has become an element of the good life and contributes to the normalization of psychoactive drug use (Elliott 2003).

Conclusion

Measham and Brain's analysis suggests that changing the role of intoxication in young people's drinking practices may be difficult, but it also suggests that possibilities exist for encouraging less-risky intoxication. Drunkenness may be celebrated as an uncontrolled state of release and liberation from norms, but in fact the young drinkers Measham and Brain (2005: 274) interviewed in Manchester aimed for a hedonistic yet bounded drinking style which could be described as a 'controlled loss of control' (see also Measham 2002). They had plans for self-regulation and management and they aimed to attain and not exceed their desired state of intoxication because of concerns such as personal safety, security, hangovers, sports and work performance (Measham and Brain 2005: 274).

The distinction between carnal and disciplined pleasure is also destabilized by the controlled hedonism found in contemporary drinking cultures. While this differentiation of pleasure is analytically useful, it tends to reproduce problematic dichotomies connected to the moderation/intoxication binary deployed by public-health discourse. Categorizing pleasure as carnal *or* disciplined places body against reason and does not capture the controlled loss of control observed in young people's leisure pursuits. The pleasures of intoxication are carnal and bodily pleasures, but they are not therefore outside the realm of discipline and management. First, as the sociological research shows, many drinkers manage their intoxication, and thus their pleasure is both carnal and disciplined. Second, in contemporary economies of consumption, carnal pleasures cannot simply be viewed as those that are transgressive, raw and outside of and resistant to social regulation. Rather, the commodification of hedonism is crucial to modern economies and therefore carnal pleasures, including those of intoxication, are deliberately managed and shaped by corporate and governmental forces. Intoxication cannot be reduced to a harm, risk or disorder, but neither should it be celebrated as an unmediated and authentic expression of libidinal energy. Like all consumptive behaviour, it is embodied, social and situational rather than an abstract and universal category with a fixed meaning.

Notes

Acknowledgements: This chapter is based on a paper presented at the *Thinking Drinking II* conference held in Melbourne, Australia, in 2006. The author would like to thank the Australian Drug Foundation for organizing the conference, and the participants for their comments.

1 Anzac Day, celebrated on 25 April, is a national day of remembrance for Australians and New Zealanders who have served and died in military operations. It specifically commemorates the Australian New Zealand Army Corps (ANZAC) Gallipoli campaign in World War I.
2 Indeed, Nicholas Emler's review of research found that engaging in physically risky pursuits such as driving under the influence of alcohol or speeding were associated with high rather than low self-esteem (2001: 59).
3 Warner's article on the 'gin epidemic' explicitly highlights its similarities to the inner-city US 'crack epidemic' of the 1980s and 1990s.

References

American Psychiatric Association (2000) *Diagnostic and Statistical Manual of Mental Disorders: DSM-IV-TR*, 4th edn, Washington, DC: American Psychiatric Association.

Beccaria, F. and Guidoni, O. (2002) 'Young people in a wet culture: Functions and patterns of drinking', *Contemporary Drug Problems*, 29(2): 305–336.

Bennett, C. and Bilardi, J. (2004) *'Is Getting Pissed Getting Pathetic?' A Report of the Joint VAADA/YACVic Youth Binge Drinking Forum*. Online, available at: www.vaada.org.au/resources/detail.chtml?filename_num=16153 (accessed 20 May 2007).

Brady, M. (2008) *First Taste: How Indigenous Australians Learned about Grog, Book 1: Aims and Ideas*, Deakin, ACT: The Alcohol Education and Rehabilitation Foundation.

Brain, K., Parker, H. and Carnwath, T. (2000) 'Drinking with design: Young drinkers as psychoactive consumers', *Drugs: Education, Prevention and Policy*, 7(1): 5–20.

Coveney, J. and Bunton, R. (2003) 'In pursuit of the study of pleasure: Implications for health research and practice', *Health*, 7(2): 161–179.

Douglas, M. (1990) 'Risk as a forensic resource', *Dadelus*, 119(4): 1–16.

Duff, C. (2004) 'Drug use as a practice of the self', *International Journal of Drug Policy*, 15: 385–393.

Elliott, C. (2003) *Better Than Well: American Medicine Meets the American Dream*, New York: W.W. Norton.

Emler, N. (2001) *Self-Esteem: The Costs and Causes of Low Self Worth*, York: York Publishing Services.

Kapferer, B. (1988) *Legends of People, Myths of State*, Washington, DC: Smithsonian Institute Press.

Lindsay, J. (2003) 'Partying hard, partying sometimes or shopping: Young workers' socializing patterns and sexual, alcohol and illicit drug risk taking', *Critical Public Health*, 13(1): 1–14.

Lindsay, J. (2006) 'A big night out in Melbourne: Drinking as an enactment of class and gender', *Contemporary Drug Problems*, 33: 29–61.

MacAndrew, C. and Edgerton, R. (1969) *Drunken Comportment: A Social Explanation*, Chicago: Aldine.

Measham, F. (2002) 'Doing gender – doing drugs: Conceptualising the gendering of drugs cultures', *Contemporary Drug Problems*, 29(2): 335–373.

Measham, F. (2004) 'The decline of ecstasy, the rise of binge drinking and the persistence of pleasure', *Probation Journal*, 51(4): 309–326.

Measham, F. and Brain, K. (2005) 'Binge drinking, British alcohol policy and the new culture of intoxication', *Crime, Media, Culture*, 1(3): 262–283.

Midford, R. (2005) 'Australia and alcohol: Living down the legend', *Addiction*, 100: 891–896.

Ministerial Council on Drug Strategy (2006a) *National Alcohol Strategy 2006–2011*, Canberra: Commonwealth of Australia.

Ministerial Council on Drug Strategy (2006b) *National Drug Strategy: Aboriginal and Torres Strait Islander Peoples Complementary Action Plan 2003–2009: Background Paper*, Canberra: Commonwealth of Australia.

Moore, D. (2006) 'Where did the pleasure go in drug discourses?', paper presented at Dangerous Consumptions IV colloquium, Australian National University, Canberra.

Mugford, S. (1993) 'Harm reduction: Does it lead where its proponents imagine?', in N. Heather, A. Wodak, E. Nadelmann and P. O'Hare (eds) *Psychoactive Drugs and Harm Reduction: From Faith to Science*, London: Whurr, pp. 21–33.

National Health and Medical Research Council (2001) *Australian Alcohol Guidelines: Health Risks and Benefits*, Canberra: Commonwealth of Australia.

O'Malley, P. and Valverde, M. (2004) 'Pleasure, freedom and drugs: The uses of pleasure in liberal governance of drug and alcohol consumption', *Sociology*, 38(1): 25–42.

Room, R. (1984) 'Alcohol control and public health', *Annual Review of Public Health*, 5: 293–317.

Room, R. (1988) 'The dialectic of drinking in Australian life: From the Rum Corps to the wine column', *Australian Drug and Alcohol Review*, 7: 413–437.

Room, R. (1998) *Controlled Drinking as a Moral Achievement and a Social Program*. Online, available at: www.doctordeluca.com/Library/AbstinenceHR/ CDasMoralAchievement98.htm (accessed 14 April 2007).

Room, R., Babor, T. and Rehm, J. (2005) 'Alcohol and public health', *The Lancet*, 365: 519–530.

Warner, J. (1994) 'In another city, in another time: Rhetoric and the creation of a drug scare in eighteenth-century London', *Contemporary Drug Problems*, 21(3): 485–511.

8 Smoking causes creative responses

On state anti-smoking policy and resilient habits

Simone Dennis

Introduction

This chapter begins with the observation that the presentation of the body as an enclosed, diagrammable and discrete biological system is a crucial element of many anti-smoking advertisements. I argue that this presentation works against several propensities of the body to move out beyond its ostensible bounds. In these propensities are grounds for asserting embodied agency against the containment of the biomedically constructed (and televised) body. These grounds are enriched by the biotechnology of cigarettes, since cigarettes offer up to the smoking person a dramatic demonstration of his or her own corporeal extension and entailment in the world. I then move to ethnographically explore the ways in which the habited past of the smoker's body is closed off in articulations of a healthy future, and how such representations may produce an ironic return to the habited body, via the cigarette and all its entailed embodied comportments.[1] Finally, I explore the ways in which the biotechnology of cigarettes disrupts the disciplined and compliant body because, in their capacity to re-temporalize the body and open it up to an unknown future, they open the body's forces onto the realm of potentiality. In this section I take two different ethnographic cases to draw out some of the potentials of smoking to open up, in the first case, an unpredictable and exciting future and, in the second, to demonstrate one of the ways in which the risky practice of smoking can be used to reduce a much more terrifying danger.

The I will exceed the I

In phenomenological tradition, one's own body is known to exceed itself, in the sense that it is not experienced as a contained entity, but rather goes out into the things of the world. The point of intersection between people and things is thus invisible to us in habitual living. Michel Polanyi (1966) argued that the points of intersection with any used object are not only routinely but *necessarily* left outside of our self-conscious attention, in order for a person to engage in any activity – speaking, walking, smoking a cigarette – in a competent manner. Merleau-Ponty's (1962) similar insight about the necessity of disattending the points at which one intersects with a world that is theoretically, but not experientially or practically, located externally to the person led him to proclaim that there is no inner person. People, rather, know themselves in the world, and *only* in the world. Such a body is pre-reflectively geared in with the world: it is a nonconscious but absently available body ordinarily 'passed over in silence' (see Sartre 1934), a body whose edges are necessarily eliminated in the ordinary course of talking, smoking, living.

Anti-smoking advertisements often draw specific attention to aspects of the smoking body, aspects that are inaccessible to the smoker in the course of 'having a fag'. These advertisements issue a kind of invitation to what Langer (1989) called the 'present body'. Present bodies invite reflection and allow persons to discover their own activity 'in shaping the world as it is discovered through our perception' (Compton 2001: 4). Present attention is drawn to the body in anti-smoking advertisements in and through the ways in which they raise self-awareness of one's own systems and separable parts of the body. To the end of self-awareness, lungs are depicted inside the body. Hearts appear as discrete organs, as do brains, throats, aorta and eyes, which all appear (diseased and damaged) in either a surgical context as an operation is underway, or outside the body and autopsy-ready, on stainless-steel trays. These separable aspects of the body are shown to belong, or at least to at one time to have belonged, inside the site of the body: a region which, as a less usually 'presently' oriented person, 'I' am unfamiliar with. The tight focusing of present attention to the unseen regions of the body brings about a view of that body as one wholly contained within, and separate from, any external world with which it might more habitually engage.

As Abram (1996) has noted, the sum total of these 'separable' and diagrammable systems or parts of the body is experientially different from the 'body subject' that Merleau-Ponty (1962) described in *Phenomenology of Perception* as the living and attentive body. Abram notes in particular that:

> This breathing body ... is very different from that complex machine whose broken parts or stuck systems are diagnosed by our medical doctors and 'repaired' by our medical technologies. Underneath the anatomized and mechanical body that we have learned to conceive ... dwells the body as it actually experiences things, this poised and animate power that initiates all our projects and suffers all our passions.
>
> (1996: 4)

Abram's insight leads me to consider the possibility that anti-smoking advertisements contain the seeds of subtle embodied resistance. This resistance is indeed subtle, in the sense that it speaks to the tendency of ordinariness, of habitualness, and, in Serres' words, to the tendency of the living body to exceed itself:

> The body goes out from the body in all senses ... the body never persists in the same plane or content but plunges and lives in a perpetual exchange, turbulence, whirlwind, circumstance. The body exceeds the body, the I surpasses the I, identity delivers itself from belonging at every instant, I sense therefore I pass, chameleon, in a variegated multiplicity.
>
> (1998: 408–409)

In such a view, the body is loathe to be located and contained within its own site – indeed, in Serres' view, such a body would be dead or 'limp', for bodies are faculties rather than things, and are only defined in sensory action. A body shown to be reduced to less may very well not recognize itself as itself, and might seek to reassert its external inclination; as Merleau-Ponty (1962) argued, in subjection, such as the reduction of the body to its biological components, the potential embedded in human agency 'goes limp'.

The fact that viewers watching these advertisements are not dead or limp goes some way to explaining why many of my own informants refused to accept that their future was indubitably one in which their own lungs wound up on a hospital table, subjected to the interested views of surgeons, coroners and public-health experts, who might make advertisements in which they featured.[2] Diprose (2008) has argued that smokers frequently refuse this future in their reassertion of an open future, but, according to Merleau-Ponty (1962), a body will also reassert its potentiality, its inclination towards its physical and social environment, when confronted with the prospect of corporeal containment (see also Serres 1982). If a body is inclined to do this as part and parcel of being an active agent in the world, then the practice of smoking cigarettes offers one particularly ready way of demonstrating a continuing inclination towards the world. Some theoreticians have even argued that smoking asserts our intertwinement with the world 'out there' in the most dramatic of ways. Katz (1999), for example, has argued that the way in which smoke marks a person's respiratory reach in the world accounts for much of the appeal of smoking.

As I have noted in my previous work on smoking (see Dennis 2006), smoke, endowed with the capacity for visually traceable travel via personal breath, can travel outbound, moving beyond the bounds of where a body, in that Kantian notion of 'receptivity' (in which a perceiving and wholly sited body remains passively receptive to the world's range of stimuli), would have to 'stay'. The fact that smokers can see that their breath escapes the sitedness of the body, as Katz (1999) argues, indicates just how much of an escape smoking actually is – so much so that our personal escapes can be visibly evidenced in a breath normally hidden from our

view. Tobacco companies have prudently imagined several appealing desti-
nations to which we might travel in these smoky outbound journeys,
including Flavour Country, and those lovely tropical islands that make up
the Menthol group. These advertisements, and indeed our own respirating
bodies, insist that we depart from the notion that our bodies are containers
(as the anti-smoking advertisements suggest). Here, the practice of smoking
offers a powerful demonstration of our entailments with the world, our
continuing life in it, and our extension out from the evidently awful confines of the naturalized body of mainstream biomedical practice, comprised
as it is of rotted lungs and choked aorta.[3]

But perhaps we should consider the redirection of ordinarily habitual
and outbounded attention to the innards and systems of the ostensibly
contained biological body. Is it really so unnatural, so horrid, to direct
attention to it? And will the body be quite as oriented as I have suggested
to an escape of its biological confines? As Lundin (1999) has pointed out,
the interior of the body is currently understood as one of the most pronounced risk fields, in stark contrast with the notion that the body is most
subject to attacks issuing from the outside, that might break through the
boundaries of the body (see Douglas 1966; Nelkin and Lindee 1995).
Lundin also notes that:

> [t]here is an extensive scholarly discussion of the significance of
> viewing one's own body and one's interior in detached segments.... In
> medical contexts, people are viewed with a medical gaze, with priority
> attached to the measurable body, while the people themselves may feel
> that they have been torn from a context.
>
> (1999: 15)

Despite recognizing the propensity of the biomedical gaze to compart-
mentalize and contain, to tear habited bodies out of their extended-into-
the-world contexts, Lundin (1999) also points out that the opportunity to
look inside the body allows her informants, who are organ-transplant
patients, to grasp and make less alien those regions: to make them 'more
their own'. While those in receipt of organs deriving from unknown others
have every reason and compulsion to bring the inner organs of the body
into their possession (not least because death might be the result if the
organs do not 'feel at home'), smokers have every reason to refuse ownership and attention to their innards.[4]

The sort of agency that Lundin (1999) argues is present in the attention
one might pay to one's own biological matter is, in fact, exactly the sort of
agency that is ostensibly available to smokers in anti-smoking discourse.
Indeed, these advertisements and the paradigm from which they issue insist
on a kind of bioethical agency that is enacted in the taking of responsibility
for one's own biological capital. As Braidotti (2007) has suggested, this
sort of agency has the capacity to force the abandonment of the naturalist

paradigm (that would reduce life to the biologically determined, and that I will discuss in detail as *zoe* in the next section). This is because embedded in this notion of agency is the idea that one will have a high degree of lucidity about one's own biological existence, which might have been priorly unknown. This capacity goes begging in anti-smoking advertisements, however, in the presentation of the smoker as irresponsible and unintelligent. Smokers are shown to have carelessly relinquished responsibility for their own biological capital. It must, therefore, be managed for them: for smokers, reaping the benefits of investment in the biological means subscribing to the flattened future body presented to them in anti-smoking advertisements and the subsequent (and somewhat ironic) relinquishment of one of the key components of agency: unpredictability. I examine this notion of unpredictability in greater detail in what follows.

To account for both of these kinds of possibilities – both the turn to and the turn away from the biological body – I return to Merleau-Ponty's view of the body, which is unrestricted in that the body is our general medium for having a world and it must be acknowledged that this world entails, at times, the restriction of the body to the actions necessary for the conservation of life. As Merleau-Ponty (1962: 146) notes, a body then 'accordingly posits around us a biological world', as it does for organ-transplant patients, and those who for other reasons must attend to the business of returning the sick or ailing body to a condition of health. But, as Merleau-Ponty also noted (1962: 146), at other times the body elaborates upon these primary actions and, 'moving from their literal to a figurative meaning, it manifests through a core of new significance; this is true of motor habits' – in which we could certainly include smoking. Smoking is significant because it allows the smoker to break through the impacts that cigarettes might have on the biological body to involve the smoker in a series of other entailments that reach out and elaborate 'primary' or basic actions – including the action of breathing. In a breath, the smoking person breathes peculiarly, and in so doing marks breath figuratively; beyond its survival at the level of biology, in this breath, the body reminds itself of its entailment with the world beyond the sited biological body. It is to the embodied manifestations beyond the primary activity of staying alive that I turn to now to explore the habited smoking body and the peculiar trust that smokers place in it, and the abandonment that smokers are required to make of it in order to participate in a healthful future, in anti-smoking advertisements.

The body will reference its embodied past to make its unpredictable future

Where I have argued in the preceding section that smoking practice itself offers a way out of the contained and systematized body that few of our number experience in the course of habitual living, Rosalyn Diprose

(2008) has argued that the practice of smoking can be understood as an ironic response to the de-temporalization to which the living body is subjected in anti-smoking advertisements. Diprose argues that a continuous progression from past to future is effected in anti-smoking advertisements. She notes that, within the paradigm of pre-emption, the advertisements present the message that health and future security will be the assured result of the cessation of the risky practice of smoking. For Diprose (2008: 143), the message 'implies the body would be thus returned to a natural order of becoming thus allowing a continuous progression from the past to the future'. Diprose's argument about the ineffectiveness of anti-smoking advertisements is based on the closing of a priorly open future that the advertisements suggest, and more particularly for the consequences this has for agency. Drawing on Merleau-Pontian phenomenology, Diprose argues that the embodied human being is at once historical and opened to an undetermined future, a multiply of potentialities. In Arendtian terms, this is human being as *bios* (as distinct from *zoe* – mere life determined by biology alone, and the forces of nature) (see Arendt 1998). *Bios* is the condition of agency, which includes the capacity to transform the past, which may result in any number of future potentialities (Diprose 2008: 146). Following Keane (2002, 2006), Diprose observes that a body subjected to a flattened and determined future will try to emerge from the sense of timelessness that such a determination imposes, to reorient itself once again to an undetermined future. She situates smoking as a social practice that precisely temporalizes the human being as *bios* – it punctuates the passing of time, with openings to an undetermined future. Diprose's focus on the re-temporalizing capacities of cigarettes has made me consider the habited body that constitutes the smoker's *past*. More specifically, it has caused me to consider what is required to be relinquished of the habited body, so that it might occupy the healthy future that is being established for it as a biological certainty in anti-smoking advertisements, if one quits the habit.

One element of embodied agency or human being as *bios* is the capacity to transform the past (Diprose 2008: 146). In current anti-smoking advertisements in Australia, the smoking person is required to abandon the smoking habits of the past body in order to inhabit a healthy future body, not, in fact, to effect a break with the past, but *in order to create an uninterrupted biological continuance with the past*. As Diprose notes, the aim embedded in anti-smoking advertisements is to connect the biological potential of the healthy past body with the biological destiny of the healthy future body, or else to connect the sickly present body with its doomed future, as a pair of lungs on the mortician's table. The requirement to abandon the habits of the past smoking body in order to accomplish the former sort of biological continuance is made plain in advertisements such as 'Everybody Knows',[5] which claims that 'everybody knows smoking causes all these diseases [including lung cancer, chronic bronchitis, throat cancer], but you *still* smoke' (emphasis added). In Quitline advertisements that immediately follow 'Everybody Knows', viewers are told that the habited smoking body can be effectively left in the past if nicotine addiction is overcome. Only when a biological body is 'freed' of nicotine dependence can it move forward to claim its biological destiny as a healthy body. Setting aside the evidently Cartesian tone of the advertisements, in which the rational mind can wrest control over the body in order to return it to its healthful biological destiny, leaving the smoking body in the past requires an unsettling disruption to the more-than-biological life of the body. The accomplishment of the biologically continuous body required in the anti-smoking advertisements equally requires the agent to draw upon their own capacities to break with the past and thus to participate in their own movement out of future potentiality to the bare life of biological certainty. In requiring smokers to enact their own capacity to break with their habited pasts, anti-smoking advertisements call upon agents to produce a body reduced to the condition of *zoe*. Here, agents may look to their habited pasts, rather than relinquish them, to reassert their agency in the face of bare life.

Something else has to happen, too, if agents are required to abandon past habited bodies in order to move into a biologically determined future. Merleau-Pontian phenomenology suggests that a body orients itself towards an open and unpredictable future with a deeply experienced past: 'perceptual life ... is subtended by an "intentional arc", which projects round about us our past, our future our human setting' (Merleau-Ponty 1962: 136). Here, a body is understood to carry forward into an open future collective history intermingled with experience of personal history, but it is also carrying with it a peculiar trust. Abandoning this trust is qualitatively different from trusting that smoking will kill you unless you give it up. I asked Nathan about his attempts at quitting. 'I don't so much buy that I'm addicted to nicotine,' he said, and continued thoughtfully:

> What I found really hard – the hardest – was that I didn't know what the hell to do with myself. You know when people say they don't know what to do with their hands? Well I didn't know what to do with my whole body. Like after dinner, which is the fag I miss the most next to the early morning one – well, all of them I missed actually – I don't go outside for that one, because I'm at home. Well, I sat in the chair where my ashtray is, and I just felt wrong. I had nothing to do with my hands. I felt a stranger in my own body. And when I'm taking a break from work. Going outside and just standing there – so not the same. And the house itself; I so miss that smell – it smells like home so much to me – they said on the Quitline that I would start to smell and taste things differently, and I wish to God I didn't. I'll always think smoking smells like home. Mum and Dad both smoked, so I think I even associate it with their house.

Nathan's comments reveal that the unspoken and unconsidered foundational trust he had priorly in his own body had been substantially shaken in his quitting attempts. As O'Neill (2009: 218) has noted, 'whatever we are bodily habituated to becomes foundational and will not usually be doubted'. Drawing on Moyal-Sharrock's (2004) discussion of 'taking things on trust', who in turn draws on Wittgenstein's (1969) distinction between rational knowing and bodily awareness, O'Neill extends this idea to distinguish between *ur*-trust, that trust developed in and through the experiencing body, and epistemic trust, which, unlike *ur*-trust, is the subject of fairly consistent questioning and critique.[6] Here, *ur*-trust is indubitable, default, the stuff of 'unconscious certainty' (see Moyal-Sharrock 2004: 197). The experienced smoking body, like other experienced habited bodies, develops an ontological security in its own bodily being in the world in and through the accumulated and confirmatory bodily experiences of being and, importantly, of being embodied as a smoking person. Cigarettes can, of course, be understood as crucial in the development of this priorly habited, unquestioned body as foundational in habited *'techniques du corps'* (or forms of bodily use) (see Mauss 1979; Jackson 1983: 334). In and through frequent interactions between body and (cigarette) object, smoking practice both creates and maintains patterns of body use; our own bodies become ingrained through our interactions with objects, including cigarettes. But there is more to it than this; there is more than bodily use involved, as smoking infiltrates bodies at the level of the senses.

As Nathan's testimony readily evidences, his unreflected, totally ordinary, processes of smelling, tasting, sitting in his chair, being at home, being himself are all inextricably intertwined with smoking. Smoking infiltrates his very 'Nathan-ness'; it makes his smelling, breathing, sitting, his sense of being at home the stuff of disregarded and unconscious embodiment. And Nathan trusts it; before he tried to quit, he did not question the surety of his sense of smell, his way of sitting, for it was beyond a shadow of a doubt. It was only when he attempted to quit (resultant of 'a bit of a health scare') that trust in his own embodied comportment was questioned, in and through the epistemological medical frame that reassessed his body for him. Despite his scare, Nathan returns to his habitual smoking past, for it is this past that allows him to conceive of his present as liveable and his future as sufficiently uncertain, to the point, at least, that it does not include the absolute certainly of lung cancer. As he himself suggested, 'I dunno if I am going to die of lung cancer, but I do know that being without smokes makes me unhappy'.

None of the things I have said in this section mean that the set of relations between ideas, experiences and bodily practices are unbreakable. People, after all, quit smoking; some people even manage to do it for good. But quitting entails a disruption not only of the relationship between ontological *ur*-trust and epistemological knowledge that ushers in the discomfort of the uncanny (see O'Neill 2009), but also between the comforting past this has created – the home of the body, if you like – and the future (according to anti-smoking advertisements, of good health and rosy prospects) – which may, in fact, be filled with the terrifying spectre of a totally unfamiliar and uninhabited non-smoking embodiment, in which even smelling is horribly unfamiliar. The trusted home of the body is pitted against the epistemic knowledge of a healthful biological body accomplished in anti-smoking advertisements and, for Nathan, his own sense of smell and his own way of sitting presented the more compelling truth. And not only this, as Diprose would have it: this smoking-derived truth is subtended by an intentional arc that opens Nathan's future to a range of potentialities over and above his imminent death from a smoking-related illness. After all, Nathan readily suggested several other ways in which he might die other than from lung cancer: he thinks he'll probably be taken down in a car accident, as he always drives too fast.[7]

The body seeks possibilities

Biotechnologies are political because they are mobilized within disciplinary regimes,

> and so participate in the reproduction of normalised, productive, compliant subjectivities that are compatible with a neoliberal political economy … but disciplinary power that renders bodies docile … does not exhaust or even best characterise, the political dimension of biotechnologies.
>
> (Diprose 2008: 145)

Here, Diprose means to suggest that biotechnologies, including cigarettes and the public-health discourse that surrounds them, can be brought into the service of interested agents, whatever else the biotechnology is meant to accomplish at the level of the cells. According to Diprose, this is because biotechnologies can be brought into the service of disciplinary power in that they can accomplish the production of the useful body (in accomplishing in and for that body a greater aptitude or capacity), but they rarely aim at obedience or compliance. Instead, they and the discourses by which they are surrounded 'aim at the enhancement of life for its own sake'. The biotechnology of cigarettes, in this view, disrupts the disciplined compliant body because, in their capacity to re-temporalize the body and open it up to an unknown future, they open the body's forces onto the realm of potentiality. As Helen Keane (2006: 107) has suggested, the 'stubborn ordinariness' of smoking suggests that the smoker is not a passive victim of addiction to a substance that will inevitably ruin one's life. Instead of inevitability, smoking 'punctuates the passing of time with openings to a different future' (Diprose 2008: 146).

I have written before about people who use smoking, and who use public-health messages about smoking, in non-compliant or even disobedient ways (see Dennis 2006). In the first of these cases, Megan used smoking to disrupt her disciplined body to open up unpredictable possibilities for casual sex with strangers (Dennis 2006: 53). During the course of that ethnographic encounter, I established that Megan used the physicality of cigarettes, in particular their length, to extend her own reach in the world. I argued that Megan effectively utilized the dissolving boundary between cigarette object and her own hand when she spoke of her attempts to 'look sexy and elegant' as she smoked. Megan said:

> 'I always smoke long cigarettes, Super Kings, and lately, I have been considering using a cigarette holder' … she looked disapprovingly at her hands. 'My hands are really pudgy, and my fingers are short and squat', she complained. 'When I hold a cigarette, like this', she said, holding up her 'smoking fingers', 'my whole arm looks longer, and I feel more elegant. It's like wearing false eyelashes, for that illusion of length'. 'What do you do with your other hand?' I asked. 'Champagne flute', she replied instantly. 'Long-stemmed'. The holding of cigarette object in the short fingers of the pudgy hand effectively extended these shortcomings into the longer reach of Megan, as the cigarette became part of fingers, the fingers part of cigarette. Megan had her longer hand.
>
> (see Dennis 2006: 53)

In that ethnographic encounter, Megan also talked about what she did with the smoke she expelled if she happened to be flirting with someone while she smoked with lengthy elegance:

> 'If I'm interested', she said, 'I like to blow my smoke up around the side of his face, like a caress'. She stroked the side of my face in an upward motion, to show me what she meant. She indicated with her fingers that the smoke trailed up beyond the face and whispered away. I asked her if it worked. 'They get the message', she replied. 'How about if you want them to leave you alone?' I asked, intrigued. 'Then I blow it straight in their face, into their eyes', she said, grinning maliciously. 'It's like giving someone a smelly slap in the face, without getting charged with assault'. 'Does anyone do it to you?', I asked. 'Yep. You can tell, if a man lets the smoke just slide out of his mouth, as opposed to blowing it out while he's perving on you or flirting with you, you can be pretty sure he wants to slide something else into you as well'.
>
> (Dennis 2006: 53)

In her involvement of cigarettes in her flirtatious practice, Megan capitalizes on their potential to disrupt compliance (including to particular standards of sexual conduct). She also rejects a future in which her body moves ever-closer to the mortician's table, and reorients it to a future where unpredictability is paramount – for Megan, there are important and immediate questions in which her smoke entails her: will I have sex tonight? With whom?

During my fieldwork, I encountered some young pregnant women who were worried about giving birth. One in particular, let us call her 'Michelle', told me about how she smoked with purpose, in order to reduce the birth weight of her baby. Here, Michelle used a biotechnology that has been specifically linked with the wreaking of havoc on the human body. When I asked her about what she knew about smoking, Michelle demonstrated that she was not ignorant of the dangers smoking presented to her body. She knew it might make her sick. She said:

> I know that smoking can give you cancer. You would have to live in a cave not to know about that. I mean, with all the ads on telly and on your pack, and so on. There was this piece in *Cosmo* or *Cleo* that also said that smoking gives you loads more wrinkles than you would get if you never done it in the first place.[8]

Clearly, Michelle knew about risks and dangers, but she also knew about the potential of smoking to reduce a risk she was presented with in her immediate future: the thought of something large emerging from her small body. Ironically, participating in smoking and its potentially damaging future led to what Michelle perceived as the reduction of risk; where anti-smoking discourse embeds having a low-birth-weight infant as a significant risk of smoking, Michelle made recourse precisely to this 'risk' to actively reduce her own risk of delivering a big baby, a prospect that loomed large in her future.[9]

Conclusion

As Lundin (1999: 8) has noted, one prominent feature of biotechnology is its capacity to get us to consider 'the boundary between focusing on the alien as a risk or as a potential'. Such an observation extends from the alien organs that Lundin's informants had to consider inserting into their bodies to validly include cigarettes. Cigarettes are situated as one biotechnology that offer to their consumers both risk and potential. As Merleau-Ponty (1962) noted, potentiality is never wholly suppressed by the threat of risk. Some smokers, at least, find potential in the practice of smoking. In being presented with the diseased systems or rotted parts in anti-smoking advertisements, which could be avoided in our submission to a biologically determined healthful future, our body, that body that initiates all our projects and suffers all our passions, might seek and, in many cases, find its escape in the comfort of a habitual and potential-expanding cigarette.

Notes

1 I have been conducting ethnographic fieldwork among smokers in Australian cities since 2004.
2 We must consider the possibility that these intentions are good and oriented towards well-being. But they still might beget resistance. Here we might consider Derrida's (2003: 94) notion that a living being will work 'to destroy its own protection'.
3 Perhaps we should consider more closely the wordlessness of such resistance; it is clearly the case that few express the view that smoke entails them in the world using words. My focus on the embodied character of lived experience reflects my conviction that analysis should be consonant with those deeply embedded practices that often remain in the realm of the unspoken. It also refuses the idea that words are always the best indicators of what is important or relevant. The wordlessness of the pleasure of smoking practice, the unarticulated pleasure of watching the smoke go out through the air and extending reach in the world, is also important.
4 However, as Nathan's case, included in the next section, suggests, there are times when the smoker wishes to know about the condition of the internal organs, if only to grant themselves license to continue smoking, secure in the knowledge that their organs have not proceeded down the path predicted for them in anti-smoking discourse.
5 Images are accompanied by Leonard Cohen's well-known lyric.
6 This distinction, between epistemic and ontological varieties of trust and knowing, does not mirror a Cartesian dualism of mind/body distinction, but refers instead to different ways of interpreting and experiencing information.
7 Diprose (2008: 143) notes that people often invoke potential deaths other than those related to smoking, as a way of re-establishing a width over the narrow course of biological life (or death) imposed in anti-smoking advertisements.
8 She knew that smoking might cause her a wrinkly face – this, too underscores Haines-Saah's point (this volume) that anti-smoking campaigns sometimes draw in appearance.
9 Anecdotal evidence like this connects with larger (pan-Western) discourses on teen mothers and moral panic (see, for example, Bell *et al.* 2009). A 2006 *Daily Mail* article declaring that UK teens were taking up smoking to reduce the possibility of delivering a large infant stirred one reader to comment that the practice was a damning insight into the ' "Vicki Pollard" infested land we live in' (*Daily Mail* 2006: 4).

References

Abram, D. (1996) *The Spell of the Sensuous: Perception and Language in a More-Than-Human World*, New York: Vintage Books.
Arendt, H. (1998) *The Human Condition*, Chicago: University of Chicago.
Bell, K., McNaughton, D. and Salmon, A. (2009) 'Medicine, morality and mothering: Public health discourses on foetal alcohol exposure, smoking around children and childhood overnutrition', *Critical Public Health*, 19(2): 155–170.
Braidotti, R. (2007) 'Bio-power and necro-politics: Reflections on an ethics of sustainability', *Springerin*. Online, available at: www.springerin.at/dyn/heft_text.php?textid=1928andlang=en (accessed June 9 2010).
Compton, J. (2001) *Embracing the Body of Culture: Understanding Cross-Cultural Psychology From the Perspective of a Phenomenology of Embodiment*. Online,

available at: http://home.earthlink.net/~rationalmystic.cultsoma.htm (accessed 10 Jun 2004).

Daily Mail (2006) 'Pregnant teens take up smoking to avoid pain of childbirth', *Mail Online*. Online, available at: www.dailymail.co.uk/news/article-408367/ Pregnant-teens-smoking-avoid-pain-childbirth.html (accessed 10 June 2010).

Dennis, S. (2006) 'Four milligrams of phenomenology: An anthrophenomenological analysis of smoking cigarettes', *Popular Culture Review Journal*, 17(1): 41–57.

Derrida, J. (2003) 'Autoimmunity: Real and imagined symbolic suicides', in G. Borradori (ed.) *Philosophy in a Time of Terror: Dialogues with Jugen Habermas and Jacques Derrida*, Chicago: University of Chicago Press, pp. 85–136.

Diprose, R. (2008) 'Biopolitical technologies of prevention', *Health Sociology Review*, 17(2): 141–150.

Douglas, M. (1966) *Purity and Danger: An Analysis of the Concepts of Pollution and Taboo*, London: Routledge and Kegan Paul.

Jackson, M. (1983) 'Thinking through the body: An essay on understanding metaphor', *Social Analysis*, 14: 127–129.

Katz, J. (1999) *How Emotions Work*, Chicago: Chicago University Press.

Keane, H. (2002) 'Smoking, addiction, and the making of time', in J.F. Brodie and M. Redfield (eds) *High Anxieties: Cultural Studies in Addiction*, Berkeley: University of California Press, pp. 119–133.

Keane, H. (2006) 'Time and the female smoker', in E. McMahon and B. Olubas (eds) *Women Making Time: Contemporary Feminist Critique and Cultural Analysis*, Perth: University of Western Australia, pp. 94–115.

Langer, M. (1989) *Merleau-Ponty's Phenomenology of Perception: A Guide and Commentary*, Tallahassee: Florida State University Press.

Lundin, S. (1999) 'The boundless body: Cultural perspectives on xenotransplantation', *Ethnos*, 64(1): 5–31.

Mauss, M. (1935 [reprinted 1979]) *Body Techniques in Sociology and Psychology: Essays by Marcel Mauss*, London: Routledge and Kegan Paul.

Merleau-Ponty, M. (1962) *Phenomenology of Perception*, trans. C. Smith, London: Routledge and Kegan Paul.

Moyal-Sharrock, D. (2004) *Understanding Wittgenstein's On Certainty*, Basingstoke: Palgrave Macmillan.

Nelkin, D. and Lindee, S. (1995) *The DNA Mystique: The Gene as a Cultural Icon*, New York: W.H. Freeman and Company.

O'Neill, K. (2009) 'Bodily knowing as uncannily canny: Clinical and ethical significance', in J. Latimer and M. Schillmeier (eds) *Un/knowing Bodies*, Hoboken: Wiley Blackwell, pp. 216–232.

Polanyi, M. (1966) *The Tacit Dimension*, New York: Doubleday.

Sartre, J.P. (1934) *L'etre et le Neant*, Paris: Gallimard.

Serres, M. (1982) *Genesis*, trans. G. James and J. Neilson, Ann Arbor: University of Michigan Press.

Serres, M. (1998) *Les Cinq Sens*, Paris: Hachette.

Wittgenstein, L. (1969) *On Certainty*, Oxford: Blackwell Publishing.

9   The sociality of smoking in the face of anti-smoking policies

Lucy McCullough

Introduction

For much of the twentieth century, cigarette smoking was an integral part of social life (Klein 1993; Berridge 1998). With the advent of cigarettes, smoking became a 'highly ritualized prop in a full set of complex social interactions' (Brandt 1998: 164). From bars, cafes and restaurants to boardrooms and bedrooms, the cigarette was a constant presence on the North American cultural landscape (Brandt 1998). By the last third of the twentieth century, smoking had infiltrated society to such an extent that when the first Surgeon-General's *Report on Smoking and Health* was released in 1964, almost half of all adult Americans were regular smokers (Brandt 1998).

Despite the abundance of medical research published since the 1960s linking smoking to lung cancer and an array of other diseases, smoking's popularity and social acceptability largely persisted until the 1980s. By the mid-1980s, however, the evidence of the negative health effects of second-hand smoke on the non-smoker transformed 'the meaning of cigarette smoke for the non-smoker from an annoyance or nuisance into a verifiable, quantifiable health risk' (Brandt 1998: 168). This gave the anti-smoking movement the evidence they needed to legitimize the prohibition of smoking in enclosed public spaces (see Bell, this volume) and so began the public-health crusade against smoking evidenced in contemporary tobacco-control policies – 'de-normalization' strategies in particular.

Although anti-smoking public-health campaigns and policies have had a measurable effect on smoking rates, these policies have directly targeted the important social value of smoking to smokers. Drawing on interviews conducted with twenty-five smokers and recent ex-smokers in Vancouver, Canada, in 2008,[1] this chapter investigates the sociality of smoking in relation to current de-normalization policies and smokers' responses to the socio-cultural framing of their smoking, both as a disease and as a pathogen.

Smoking: addiction or choice?

While the current anti-smoking movement may have particular vigour and strength, disdain for smoking hardly began in the twentieth century. Smoking has 'been greeted with hostility, in varying degrees, for five hundred years' (Sullum 1998: 16). Much of this opposition was based on the perceived tension between the addictive nature of tobacco and the self-control necessary to maintain socially acceptable smoking patterns. In the Victorian era, arguments against smoking were based on tobacco's violation of 'liberal preoccupations with self-possession and rationality' (Rudy 2005: 7). At the same time, those smokers with the ability to withstand their desires and control their behaviour were considered to have moral fortitude. Indeed, more than any other 'consuming ritual', smoking held particular liberal symbolism (Rudy 2005: 7; see also Room, this volume, for a similar discussion on the values and morality attributed to controlled drinking). Political theorist Anthony Arblaster (as quoted in Rudy 2005: 9) argued that:

> According to 18th- and 19th-century liberal views, the rational individual 'is not the one who merely *uses* reason to guide and assist his desires. He is the man who through reason liberates himself from the tyranny of appetite and desire'. Even in this period there was an awareness of tobacco's 'tyranny of appetite and desire', but its seemingly benign effects in comparison to alcohol or drugs meant it constituted a surmountable, though not insignificant, risk and thus a particularly meaningful demonstration of self-control.

The ability of people to demonstrate self-control over smoking is indicative of a general difficulty that persists to this day in fitting smoking into a disease model of addiction that is more easily typified by other substances such as alcohol (Jellinek 1946, 1960). The criteria for addiction under a disease and dependency model include physiological symptoms of withdrawal and tolerance, psychological dependence and compulsion, and an apparent lack of control over this process (WHO 1992; APA 1994; Room 2003). As Robin Room (2003) points out, these criteria reflect a European/Western privileging of medical or 'scientific' explanations of human problems, and suggest addiction is a kind of 'secular possession' that takes over the person. Losing control is particularly problematic in a Western European context because it poses a threat to one's wealth and autonomy, and thus to their sustained consumption (Room, this volume). Smoking, then, presents itself as the hero in Western self-focused consumerist culture because smokers can be 'chronic' consumers yet remain economically and socially productive and in control.

People *do* demonstrate control over their smoking by choosing when and where it is appropriate to smoke, and often do *not* demonstrate a progressive increase in number of cigarettes smoked per day (Gillies and Willig 1997). In fact, for many smokers, smoking is an adaptive purposeful behaviour that provides moments of rest and solitude in an otherwise hectic and burdensome life (see Graham 1993, 1994, on the functionality of some women's smoking). Smokers in general do not seem to be driven to pathological levels of physical dependence, and likely do not experience a never-ending path in search of 'organismic wholeness, vitality, and a secure fund of personally relevant meaning' as readily as addicts of 'harder' substances (Saleebey 1985: 19). For these reasons, tobacco has historically been treated as quite distinct from alcohol and other drugs at a policy level, and it was only in the 1990s that tobacco, alcohol and illicit drugs began to be considered together under one scientific paradigm of addiction (Berridge 1998).

Yet, despite the incorporation of tobacco into an addictions paradigm, important differences continue to exist between policy approaches to tobacco and other drugs. Current approaches to addiction (particularly in Canada) generally focus on de-stigmatizing substance use in the hopes of lessening barriers to a range of health services. Recent policies are even incorporating harm-reduction approaches to encourage safe use of drugs and ameliorate their negative health effects (Bell *et al.* 2010b). Tobacco de-normalization policies, on the other hand, seek to stigmatize smoking and remove it from the public realm through a number of strategies, including location and point-of-sale restrictions and public-health media campaigns on the dangers of second-hand smoke (Bell *et al.* 2010b). Moreover, while policy-makers insist that the targets of de-normalization policies are the tobacco industry and smoking, not the smoker, recent observers have noted that these strategies have fostered a social transformation that appears to involve the active stigmatization of smokers (Bayer and Stuber 2006; Bayer 2008; Bell *et al.* 2010a, 2010b).

Today, smokers are often caught between societal conceptions of smoking as an addiction and their own personal experiences of tobacco. For example, in qualitative interviews with working-class women smokers, Gillies and Willig (1997) noted inconsistencies in the addictions discourse the women tended to use. Women constructed their smoking within an addiction framework, describing loss of control over the compulsion to smoke and fear of withdrawal, but at the same time described their ability to employ personal agency and control by abstaining or quitting if or when necessary. In particular, the women noted their ability to moderate their smoking behaviours in situations where smoking was prohibited.

Smokers I have interviewed express similar inconsistencies. Bill, an HIV+ smoker in his late fifties living on social assistance, saw smoking as a final freedom and pleasure, and simultaneously invoked an addictions discourse to defend it:

> I mean losing so many freedoms in our society today, like you know, like I'm treated, I think unfairly, you know, moving back to the city

and going through what I have to go through with housing issues and trying to get employment again where I'm qualified and this and that. So in losing some of my personal identity and personal freedoms I feel that, hey, smoking is my issue, my freedom, you know, I'm addicted. I'll protect it.

Bill's statement – 'smoking is my issue, my freedom, you know, I'm addicted' – reveals the paradox of agency inherent in the disease model of addiction (Valverde 1998). On the one hand, his smoking is an autonomous expression of his freedom to smoke; on the other hand, he further legitimizes his smoking by invoking a disease model of addiction which suggests that he is powerless over it.

Smokers often describe their smoking in ways that do not fit a deterministic addictions framework. In the following exchange, Musad, a smoker in his mid-twenties, indicated considerable flexibility in his tobacco use:

LM: So for you it's the context of drinking and being social that just makes it, yeah.

MUSAD: Yeah, it skyrockets from there.

LM: Skyrockets. Okay. Okay. So how would you classify your smoking then? Would you say you're like a light smoker, a medium smoker, a social smoker? Like how would you?

MUSAD: I guess I'm a light smoker but it can just jump from that to a heavy smoker, right?

LM: Right. But sort of overall you feel you're a light smoker.

MUSAD: Like tonight, say if I was drinking and partying tonight, I could be a heavy smoker tonight.

In this exchange, I am pushing Musad to characterize his smoking status more generally (e.g. heavy, light, social, etc.). However, he resists categorization and insists that his smoking status changes depending on the context. For example, he could be a heavy smoker when 'drinking and partying', but does not consider this his stable smoking pattern. Musad is like many smokers and drug users whose patterns of use are socially and contextually embedded. Unfortunately, and erroneously, the context and circumstances of tobacco consumption are neglected in current behavioural epidemiological strategies employed in counting smokers and examining causes of smoking behaviour. As Mair (this volume) describes, the neglect of context is due in large part to the fact that behavioural epidemiology has simply extended the logic of clinical reasoning, operating on the assumption that analyses of what 'causes' an individual to smoke can be modelled on the causal relationship that connects smoking to lung cancer. Social-constructionist models of addiction posit that smoking severity and patterns are context-dependent and, counter to deterministic disease models of addiction, describe addiction as an adaptive, fluid and 'complex social process that is inherently relational' (Graham *et al.* 2008: 122; see also Peele 1990). In order to understand the causes of smoking and experience of smokers, we must move away from simplistic and totalizing categories of 'smoker' or 'non-smoker', 'alcoholic' or 'controlled drinker', to focus on substance use in context (see Mair, this volume).

The inadequacies of existing models of addiction become starkly apparent in the context of 'social smokers', who describe sociality as the defining feature of their habit. Today, the term 'social smoker' is most commonly used to refer to young adults who smoke non-daily, mainly in social contexts, and are not (*yet*) physiologically dependent on nicotine (Levinson *et al.* 2007; see also Moran 2004; Waters *et al.* 2006; Kelly 2009 for definitions of social smokers). Social smokers are seen to be young because the idea is that they will invariably progress to full-blown nicotine dependence. While there has been some interest over the past few years in characterizing and defining 'social smokers' (e.g. Moran 2004; Levinson *et al.* 2007), the term often appears in quotation marks (e.g. Kelly 2009) as a problematized category. For example, in Levinson *et al.*'s (2007) study on smoking amongst college students, the students who smoked were first either categorized as 'deniers' (did not self-identify as a smoker) or 'admitters' (did self-identify as a smoker). Then, those who called themselves 'social smokers' were identified within these groups. Levinson *et al.*'s (2007) use of the language of 'admitters' and 'deniers' invokes an underlying disease-model of addiction, suggesting there are but two categories of smokers: those who are afflicted with the disease and know it and those who are afflicted and deny it. The social smoker 'category' is highly incompatible with current conceptions of smoking as an addiction because social smokers seem to maintain a low socially embedded consumption rate over a long period of time.

Although public health is only just beginning to grapple with the apparent stability of the social smoking status (see Schane *et al.* 2009), since the 1970s, the tobacco industry has recognized and researched social smokers as a *stable* and valid category of users that embodied the 'social benefits' of smoking (Schane *et al.* 2009: 125). Public-health and tobacco-control researchers, on the other hand, have traditionally conceptualized social smoking as a 'transient behaviour associated with smoking initiation or cessation' (Schane *et al.* 2009: 124) in line with a disease model of addiction. However, social smokers have recently become a focus in tobacco-control and epidemiological research – not because they defy the assumed progression of addiction from occasional user to habitual dependent addict, but because their 'denial' (of their addiction and its health risks) poses a problem to public health's ability to identify, count and intervene with smokers. In addition, the view of social smokers as a transient category is perceived to have turned attention away from the potential role of smoke-free policies in getting this group to quit (Schane *et al.* 2009).[2]

The sociality of smoking

As the accounts of social smokers suggest, sociality is intrinsic to cigarette smoking. Indeed, its rise in popularity is largely a result of its role in the First and Second World Wars as a social and psychological consolation in times of stress.[3] As Bill, a smoker in his late-fifties, notes, 'I was four years in the Canadian Army. What's a more social thing when you're sitting around having a smoke break? ... You just, it's a social thing, it's similarity.'

Smoking, as experienced by many smokers, is a social tool which provides opportunities for conversation and connection. Dennis (2006) draws a parallel between the dissolvability of smoke and the social boundaries between people, saying, 'If smoking were to be theorized through smell, we might draw different kinds of attention to smoke's capacity to dissolve existing connections, and to dissolve boundaries between persons' (2006: 51). Smokers often highlight this aspect of their habit. As Wade, a smoker in his late-twenties, notes:

> You actually are often, especially, like, in social settings, you're often talking to complete strangers through the smoking. And I think part of it is a psychological attachment to the – connecting the smoking to the social interactions and that. Even sometimes bringing us closer to our fellow man and woman that we could often be afraid of.

The image of the intermingling plumes of smoke between people provides a visual metaphor for the inherent sociality of smoking and the pleasures and functions it entails. The brevity, accessibility and minimal but immediate psychobiological effects of smoking can facilitate interpersonal connectedness and can provide easily navigable delimitations to new social interactions (Keane 2002). For example, 'asking "have you a lighter?" of a group of persons unknown to you in the pub might lead any place' (Dennis 2006: 50), while the finishing of a cigarette provides parties with clearly identifiable times at which they can leave uncomfortable or unfamiliar social settings or interactions.

The social features of smoking are also highlighted in discussions of smoking on chat-room -style websites. For example, 'FreeState' says:

> I'm a former smoker. Smoking has a lot of benefits. As a former smoker here are the benefits I miss most:
>
> * Smoking after eating – it's better than dessert.
> * The smell of smoke (I love it, always have).
> * Decreased appetite when smoking (really helped keep the weight off).
> * *The sociality of smoking in groups.*

I could go on and on – but to say there is no other purpose than to cause disease would be about as big a lie as saying we went into Iraq for Osama.

(Democratic Underground 2008, emphasis added)

The tobacco-control movement and anti-smoking public-health agendas have polarized the issue of smoking in the public realm and research community (see Bell, this volume). On the pro-tobacco-control side, all smoking is seen as pathological and dangerous, and any dissent from this position is increasingly being discredited as a denial of the harms of smoking. This polarization is evident between FreeState's position and the type of responses it generated. The above statement met with fervent disagreement. Other bloggers said that the benefits of smoking noted by FreeState were 'not useful' and were 'excuses for addiction'. Their opposition demonstrates the extent to which the addiction framework has been taken up by the general public, in this case bloggers, in the context of tobacco use. FreeState's critics echo standard tobacco-control positions that do not accept any reason, place or time for smoking. On the other side, the blogger's chosen name – FreeState – reflects an anti-nanny-state sentiment similar to those critical of current public-health tobacco-control policies and echoed by other smokers (see Bell *et al.* 2010a).

Ex-smokers often describe the 'sociality of smoking' as one of the things they miss most about smoking. Many lament the changes in their social circle that quitting smoking commonly necessitates. Louise, a forty-eight-year-old recent ex-smoker, identifies the changes in her patterns of socializing as being among the most difficult to deal with. She says:

I mean all my friends are smokers, despite that I'm not. And it's a little bit of a difficult situation because they're going out on the balcony to smoke. Let's say if I have some people at my place, I'm staying inside because I'm not a smoker. They're on the balcony smoking, let's say two of them, and meanwhile I'm inside by myself. So, you know, that's difficult. Now that I'm not in that social circle kind of thing.

The social changes resulting from quitting are often noted in the quitting literature and websites. Both the smoking-cessation support communities and the alcohol-recovery communities highlight the importance of building new social groups with non-users. In the case of Alcoholics Anonymous, developing a sober community is a therapeutic endeavour away from the 'egoistic individualism' that is considered in AA to be part of alcoholism (Room 1993: 167). One self-declared 'long-term habitual, addicted, dedicated smoker' even advises to 'divorce your friends for a year' in order to quit smoking (Quit Smoking Methods 2007).[4]

There is a loss of identity that was once exercised through smoking interactions. However, the implications of this social loss have rarely been considered beyond the risk it poses to potentiate relapse. I propose that the social aspect of smoking may predict or moderate someone's smoking career to the same extent, and maybe even more, than their level of physical dependence and addiction. Interestingly, even those ex-smokers and smokers who support and see the benefits of anti-smoking policies struggle with these changes. Louise, though strong in her resolve not to smoke, talked at length about how it is difficult now to be with the 'cooler people' she would like to hang around with. She says:

> And also like, you know, at work, you know, some of the cooler people, and the people you like to hang around with, they're all, although we don't have a chance to talk during our break, they're downstairs smoking. And I'll be upstairs let's say maybe on the computer, making phone calls or talk – you know what I mean? So that part's difficult. I'm still struggling with that after a year.... I'm not, you know I'm still having great difficulty with, but I have that will-power that I won't go down there and join them, yeah.

Younger smokers today, particularly those among the white Canadian middle-class, did not experience smoking as part of mainstream consuming rituals. Yet, the sociality of smoking continues to have an allure for adolescents and young adults.[5] According to Jackie, a twenty-two-year-old recent ex-smoker:

LM: Why do you think you became a regular smoker?

JACKIE: Why I think? I identified with the smoker, you know, until recently.... Yeah, it was a social thing at the same time. You know, I was like 'Let's go for a smoke.' 'Oh yeah!' Like when you're at school, you know, you have the smokers' corner and you know, you attract smokers, and it's so much easier to be social with someone who smokes.... So it's a very socially ... because I couldn't see myself as a non-smoker, a non-smoker I associated with someone who I wasn't, which is silly, but I think not directly focusing or thinking from the top of my head. Like that kind of thing, now I think back on it, I associated with the image of a smoker rather than a cigarette.... Yeah, so it was the jocks and cheerleaders and those people who played volleyball or something like that, you know, but I wasn't. And so there was another crowd of us that smoked cigarettes in the corner and philosophize about life and like, you know, I was that person. I was just 'Life sucks and this is why' as I, like, drag my cigarette (laughs).

Jackie, like Louise, speaks to the unique social and identity-forming interactions smoking facilitates. Jackie's statement: 'I associated with the image of a smoker rather than a cigarette', makes it clear that her identity as a smoker was more than the physical rewards of smoking. Smoking was a symbol of the 'philosophers' and their shared social identity. Here, Jackie and her friends are simultaneously achieving youth-developmental tasks of bonding and individuation as philosophers (not jocks, cheerleaders, etc.). The sociality of smoking, especially for youth, may be construed as 'peer pressure', which is always framed in entirely negative terms as a factor leading to the uptake of smoking. However, given the social nature of human beings, 'peer pressure' may serve a functional and welcome role for smokers.

Smoking de-normalization policies: transforming the social into the anti-social

Early public-health campaigns starting in the 1960s focused on educating smokers about its negative health impacts and implementing age restrictions on the purchase of cigarettes (Berridge 1998). Over time, particularly with research linking second-hand smoke to health problems, public-health messaging and anti-smoking policies have become more aggressive, invasive and directed towards the rights of non-smokers. The explicitly stated intent and effect of these policies, known as 'de-normalization' strategies, was to push smoking into a socially unacceptable realm (see Bell *et al.* 2010a, 2010b).

Smoking de-normalization strategies were pioneered in the state of California. The California Department of Health Services (1998: 3) states that: 'the goal of this "social norm change" approach is to indirectly influence current and potential future tobacco users by creating a social milieu and legal climate in which tobacco becomes less desirable, less acceptable, and less accessible.' Canada quickly followed suit, and in 1999 adopted de-normalization policies as the fourth pillar of its National Tobacco Control Strategy (Steering Committee of the National Strategy to Reduce Tobacco Use in Canada 1999). The strategy states:

> Denormalization activities are important because they may help to develop a set of values and behaviours that bring the whole community together to reinforce desirable behaviour and attitudes. It can help to make tobacco use an issue of community concern, rather than just an issue for those using the products. Secondly, it can help ensure that people behave in appropriate ways – including making efforts to quit – without the need for a lot of policing or enforcement.
>
> (1999: 25)

Fundamental to these policies is an attempt to use the sociality of smoking against the smoker. As Brandt (1998: 174) notes: 'the social aspects of smoking so critical to its popularity in the 20th century such as social conformity and peer pressure, were now employed to limit smoking.' Thus, an intrinsically social activity for much of the twentieth century was now defined as intrinsically anti-social. Through de-normalization policies, non-smokers are encouraged to 'act as an agent of enforcement' (1998: 174), and they are exhorted to 'not suffer or allow a person to smoke' (City of Vancouver 2008: 5) in any of the areas specified by non-smoking by-laws and legislation (see also City of White Rock 2008).

Many of the smokers interviewed in the Vancouver study have experienced these policy changes first-hand (see Bell *et al.* 2010a). Within their lifetime they have been first encouraged to smoke as though it were a part of normal adult life, developed the habit in a smoker-friendly environment, and have then been faced with increasing anti-smoking policies and stigma against their smoking. Mark, a forty-seven-year-old smoker, expressed his sense of embarrassment and shame over smoking. He says:

MARK: Yeah. Smoking is always an embarrassment.
LM: Do you have smoking friends?
MARK: Yes, yes I do. Yeah, so I know who they are and I can. It's just socially unacceptable, I find. It's just a dirty little thing.

Another participant, Mary, a fifty-year-old smoker, did not feel comfortable smoking anywhere in public anymore and only smoked 'in my own backyard'. By eliminating the social aspects of smoking, smokers are forced to re-cast their smoking solely as an addiction, with disempowering implications on the smokers' feelings of control over the habit (Gillies and Willig 1997; Thompson *et al.* 2007; Thompson *et al.* 2009). As Robert Castel (1991: 298) notes, 'The iatrogenic aspects of prevention are always operative even when it is consumption of such "suspect" products as alcohol or tobacco which is under attack'.

Yet, the social aspects of smoking persist in the face of anti-smoking policies and may even be heightened for some smokers in spite of (and perhaps because of) the increasingly hostile responses that smoking elicits. As Thompson *et al.* (2007: 509) state: 'while being cast as an outsider may stimulate behaviour change in order to fit in with dominant conceptions of "good citizenship", it may also give rise to active resistance which is not the desired response of anti-smoking campaigns.' As anti-smoking policies become increasingly strict, the shared identity among smokers deepens, as does their sense of camaraderie. Referring back to the connection between soldiering and smoking, some smokers today appear to feel like guerrilla fighters against a war on tobacco. Furthermore, as smoking is made synonymous with social deviance, smokers adopt and may even embrace an 'outsider identity' (Becker 1963). As Pete, a smoker in his mid-twenties, notes:

I mean, since smokers have been so ostracized I find there's a real camaraderie there, like when you're at the bar and people say, 'Oh, let's go out for a smoke', then that's actually more tempting because you know that's when the really interesting conversation is going to be, is out having a cigarette, you know, with a buddy, right.

Smoking has moved from being a shared activity in normal social circles to smokers now having a 'shared sense of solidarity in their forced retreat from the inside environs' (Kelly 2009: 574). As a smoker in the Vancouver study said, 'The pariahs are out there.' The camaraderie between smokers is one of the unintended consequences of tobacco-control policies and serves to reinforce smoking identities and behaviours. Indeed, although the focus of little study, some research has found that increased stigmatization actually reinforces continued smoking in certain populations. According to Thompson *et al.* (2007: 508), 'The increasing stigmatization of those who continue to smoke, coupled with the spatial segregation of poor and minority populations, may compound to produce "smoking islands" that may serve to reinforce rather than discourage continued smoking'. Ironically, de-normalization policies may serve to entrench the very practice they are attempting to discourage.

Conclusion

In this chapter, I have presented the valued social aspects of smoking, which are integral to both its rise in popularity as a drug over the course of the twentieth century and the narratives of contemporary smokers. In so doing, I have critiqued popular and biomedical nosologies of addiction which are confined to individuals' psychological and neuro-physiological processes. As I have shown, smokers' accounts of their 'habit' demonstrate their ambivalent engagement with the concept of addiction and the context-bound nature of much smoking. Indeed, a certain sub-group of smokers – social smokers – resist being put into a deterministic disease model of addictions altogether by smoking in an infrequent, controlled, socially and contextually bound way (e.g. at parties only).

In recent years, the *sociality* of smoking has become the target of a particularly stigmatizing and exclusionary group of 'de-normalization' policies, which emphasize protecting the rights of non-smokers in indoor and outdoor public spaces. Ironically, this policy approach of altering the context and the sociality of smoking may serve to entrench the very practice it is attempting to quell. While such policies may encourage many smokers to quit, I have shown that for at least some of those who continue to smoke, the 'de-normalization' environment serves to bind them together in solidarity with other smokers.

Notes

1 This was a pilot study funded by the Canadian Institutes of Health Research and led by Kirsten Bell that broadly explored the impact of tobacco-control policies

on smokers in Vancouver, Canada. Interviews were conducted over a seven-month period between September 2008 and March 2009. Many smokers talked about feelings of social exclusion, discrimination, self-reproach and powerlessness in quitting (see Bell *et al.*, 2010a and 2010b).

2 There is some evidence to suggest that social smokers might be more readily induced to quit through messages focused on the dangers associated with second-hand smoke, since social smokers are generally not concerned about their own health or addiction potential (see Philpot *et al.* 1999; Schane *et al.* 2009).

3 Tobacco companies such as Lucky Strike and Bull Durham were major contributors to America's military efforts in both world wars. Support of America's war efforts and of American tobacco thus become closely linked (Sullum 1998; Cordry 2001). As Klein (1993: 3) writes: 'Cigarette smoking during wartime and depression was not merely approved as a pleasure but viewed almost as a duty that owed to the principle of camaraderie and to the requirements of consolation in the face of tragedy.' Tobacco's successful alignment with the war effort was also due to smoking's ability to provide brief and accessible time-outs with minor yet pleasant neuro-physiological stimulation (see Keane 2002 for a discussion of smoking and the 'making of time'). By the time of the Vietnam War, smoking had become closely associated with soldiering.

4 There are numerous smoking-cessation websites that provide tips and incentives for quitting. The advice to 'divorce your friends for year' can be found on the website Quit Smoking Methods: Hundreds of Secrets Used by Real Smokers to Kick the Habit (Quit Smoking Methods 2007).

5 The highest rates of smoking in Canada are among young adults aged 20–24 (see Health Canada 2008).

References

American Psychiatric Association (1994) *Diagnostic and Statistical Manual of Mental Disorders*, 4th edn, Washington, DC: American Psychiatric Association.

Bayer, R. (2008) 'Stigma and the ethics of public health: Not can we but should we', *Social Science and Medicine*, 67: 463–472.

Bayer, R. and Stuber, J. (2006) 'Tobacco control, stigma, and public health: Rethinking the relations', *American Journal of Public Health*, 96(1): 47–50.

Becker, H.S. (1963) *Outsiders: Studies in the Sociology of Deviance*, London: Free Press.

Bell, K., McCullough, L., Salmon, A. and Bell, J. (2010a) ' "Every space is claimed": Smokers' experiences of tobacco denormalisation', *Sociology of Health and Illness*, 32(6): 1–16.

Bell, K., Salmon, A., Bowers, M., Bell., J. and McCullough, L. (2010b) 'Smoking, stigma and tobacco "denormalization": Further reflections on the use of stigma as a public health tool', *Social Science and Medicine*, 70: 795–799.

Berridge, V. (1998) 'Science and policy: The case of postwar British smoking policy', in S. Lock, L.A. Reynolds and E.M. Tansey (eds) *Ashes to Ashes: The History of Smoking and Health*, Amsterdam: Rodopi, pp. 143–162.

Brandt, A.M. (1998) 'Blow some my way: Passive smoking, risk and American culture', in S. Lock, L.A. Reynolds and E.M. Tansey (eds) *Ashes to Ashes: The History of Smoking and Health*, Amsterdam: Rodopi, pp. 164–191.

California Department of Health Services, Tobacco Control Section (1998) *A Model for Change: The California Experience in Tobacco Control*, Sacramento: California Department of Health Services.

Castel, R. (1991) 'From dangerousness to risk', in G. Burchell, C. Gordon and P. Miller (eds) *The Foucault Effect: Studies in Governmentality*, Chicago: University of Chicago Press, pp. 281–298.

City of Vancouver (2008) *Health By-Law No. 9535*, Vancouver: City of Vancouver.

City of White Rock (2008) *The Corporation of the City of White Rock Bylaw 1858*, White Rock: City of White Rock.

Cordry, H.V. (2001) *Tobacco: A Reference Handbook*, Santa Barbara: ABC-Clio Inc.

Democratic Underground (2008) 'Is there a hidden agenda in the current anti-smoking craze?' *Democratic Underground*. Online, available at: www.democraticunderground.com/discuss/duboard.php?az=view_allandaddress=364x1541667 (accessed 30 May 2009).

Dennis, S. (2006) 'Four milligrams of phenomenology: An anthrophenomenological analysis of smoking cigarettes', *Popular Culture Review*, 15(4): 41–57.

Gillies, V. and Willig, C. (1997) '"You get the nicotine and that in your blood": Constructions of addiction and control in women's accounts of cigarette smoking', *Journal of Community and Applied Social Psychology*, 7: 285–301.

Graham, H. (1993) *When Life's a Drag: Women, Smoking and Disadvantage*, London: HMSO/Department of Health Publications.

Graham, H. (1994) 'Surviving by smoking', in S. Wilkinson and C. Kitzinger (eds) *Women and Health: Feminist Perspectives*, London: Taylor and Francis, pp. 102–123.

Graham, M., Young, R., Valach, L. and Wood, R.A. (2008) 'Addiction as a complex social process: An action theoretical perspective', *Addiction Research and Theory*, 16(2): 121–133.

Health Canada (2008) *Canadian Tobacco Use Monitoring Survey*. Online, available at: www.hc-sc.gc.ca/hc-ps/tobac-tabac/research-recherche/stat/index-eng.php#ctums (accessed 24 June 2008).

Jellinek, E.M. (1946) 'Phases in the drinking history of alcoholics', *Quarterly Journal of Studies on Alcohol*, 7: 1–88.

Jellinek, E.M. (1960) *The Disease Concept of Alcoholism*, New Brunswick: Hillhouse Press.

Keane, H. (2002) 'Smoking, addiction, and the making of time', in J.F. Brodie and M. Redfield (eds) *High Anxieties: Cultural Studies in Addiction*, Berkeley: University of California Press, pp. 119–133.

Kelly, B.C. (2009) 'Smoke-free air policy: Subcultural shifts and secondary health effects among club-going young adults', *Sociology of Health and Illness*, 31(4): 569–582.

Klein, R. (1993) *Cigarettes are Sublime*, London: Picador.

Levinson, A.H., Campo, S., Gascoigne, J., Jolly, O., Zakharyan, A. and Vu Tran, Z. (2007) 'Smoking, but not smokers: Identity among college students who smoke cigarettes', *Nicotine and Tobacco Research*, 9(8): 845–852.

Moran, S. (2004) 'Social smoking among US college students', *Pediatrics*, 114(4): 1028–1034.

Peele, S. (1990) 'Behavior in a vacuum: Social-psychological theories of addiction that deny the social and psychological meaning of behaviour', *Journal of Mind and Behaviour*, 11(3): 393–399.

Philpot, S.J., Ryan, S.A., Torre, L.E., Wilcox, H.M., Jalleh, G. and Jamrozik, K.

(1999) 'Effect of smoke-free policies on the behaviour of social smokers', *Tobacco Control*, 8: 278–281.

Quit Smoking Methods (2007) *Multiple Steps For Quitting Smoking: Divorce Your Smoking Friends*. Online, available at: www.quitsmokingmethods.com/multiple-steps-for-quitting-smoking/divorce-your-smoking-friends.htm (accessed 30 April 2010).

Room, R. (1993) 'Alcoholics Anonymous as a social movement', in B. McCrady and W.R. Miller (eds) *Research on Alcoholics Anonymous: Opportunities and Alternatives*, Piscataway: Rutgers Center of Alcohol Studies, pp. 167–187.

Room, R. (2003) 'The cultural framing of addiction', *Janus Head*, 6(2): 221–234.

Rudy, J. (2005) *The Freedom to Smoke: Tobacco, Consumption and Identity*, Montreal and Kingston: McGill-Queen's University Press.

Saleebey, D. (1985) 'A social psychology perspective on addiction: Themes and dis-harmonies', *Journal of Drug Issues*, 15(1): 17–28.

Schane, R.E., Glantz, S.A. and Ling, P.M. (2009) 'Social smoking implications for public health, clinical practice and intervention research', *American Journal of Preventive Medicine*, 37(2): 124–131.

Steering Committee of the National Strategy to Reduce Tobacco Use in Canada (1999) *New Directions for Tobacco Control in Canada: A National Strategy*, Ottawa: Health Canada.

Sullum, J. (1998) *For Your Own Good: The Anti-Smoking Crusade and the Tyranny of Public Health*, New York: Free Press.

Thompson, L., Barnett, J.R. and Pearce, J. (2009) 'Scared straight? Fear-appeal anti-smoking campaigns, risk, self-efficacy and addiction', *Health, Risk and Society*, 11(2): 181–196.

Thompson, L., Pearce, J. and Barnett, J.R. (2007) 'Moralising geographies: Stigma, smoking islands and responsible subjects', *Area*, 39(4): 508–517.

Valverde, M. (1998) *Diseases of the Will: Alcohol and the Dilemmas of Freedom*, Cambridge: Cambridge University Press.

Waters, K., Harris, K., Hall, S., Nazir, N. and Waigandt, A. (2006) 'Characteristics of social smoking among college students', *Journal of American College Health*, 55(3): 133–139.

World Health Organization (1992) *The ICD-10 Classification of Mental and Behavioural Disorders: Clinical Descriptions and Diagnostic Guidelines*, Geneva: World Health Organization.

10 In praise of hunger

Public health and the problem of excess

John Coveney

Introduction

The idea of, and resistance to, the notion of 'excess' is now embedded in the area of public health. The problem of excess living is the most useful way of conceptualizing this. It underpins many of the policies aimed at addressing chronic diseases common in developed countries where the so-called 'good life' has led to health problems that are prevalent in the affluent world. While acknowledging that access to certain resources (e.g. enough food, clean water, adequate shelter) is important to establishing good health, there is a belief that more resources do not necessarily lead to better health. There comes a point beyond which more food, more luxuries, more leisure and other trappings of wealth can be harmful to health (Powles 2001). The problem of having too much is not merely an individual health problem, however. Public health has been quick to demonstrate that living excessively also has implications for the health of the environment, where, for example, eating too much is said to sustain a food supply that gives rise to greenhouse gases, some of which (for example, methane and nitrous oxide) are much more potent than carbon dioxide (CO2) (McMichael *et al.* 2007). Thus, it is proposed that profligate lifestyles lead not only to health problems for people, but also consume the Earth's resources and, in so doing, contribute to climate change (Friel *et al.* 2009).

The pleasures associated with an affluence lifestyle are also well recognized to be problematic for public health, with many campaigns exhorting the public to rein in excess and moderate consumption of pleasurable foods, usually those containing fat, sugar or salt (Crotty 1995). For many years in public health there has been a message of moderation: eat moderately, drink modestly and be aware of measured amounts. However, more recently there is a rising concern that moderation is simply not enough to make a difference in terms of overall health. Complete abstinence, in some cases, is the only answer. For example, in Australia, pregnant women, who previously were recommended to drink moderately, are now advised to avoid all alcohol during pregnancy (National Health and Medical Research

Council 2009). In other areas, even if complete abstinence is not openly endorsed, then certainly a discourse of frugality is encouraged in order to balance the excesses of modern life.

Looking more closely at public-health discourses, it is clear that the problems of excess food, excess alcohol, excess sedentary behaviour, etc. are, in fact, proxies for a much greater excess. Living and consuming in the twenty-first century in a developed economy (that is, a capitalist society) is seen to be at the heart of the problem. Indeed, late or advanced capitalism is itself regarded to be the target, with many examples proposed of the ways in which modern Western societies have allowed, even encouraged, individuals to run out of control, whether this is with excess eating, binge-drinking or even financial extravagance, as in the case of the 2008–2009 economic crisis fuelled by individuals encouraged to borrow beyond their means (Stiglitz 2010). LeBesco (2004) goes further by asking whether the body seen to result from excess – the fat body – can be imagined as a failed, unproductive citizen: is it a symbol of the limits of hard work and individual achievement? Is it a sign of the failure of the American Dream, because it is clear evidence that we cannot always get what we want?

The public-health antidote to this excessive lifestyle is one of thrifti-ness, a lifestyle which is pared back to essentials and minimizes excess. It is the move towards parsimony that is the focus of this chapter. Using examples drawn from public-health nutrition, it will be argued that there is now an explicit and organized backlash against the life of luxury and excess. This movement finds hubris reckless in terms of health, but also feckless in terms of the moral fortitude needed to be a wholesome citizen. The tendency towards thrift is not new to public health, however (Coveney 1999). Indeed, the field of nutritional science was first legiti-mized in the nineteenth century through an endeavour to encourage a form of nutritional reductionism that emphasized eating for economic reasons, rather than enjoyment, taste or any other more sensuous pleas-ures (Pollan 2008).

Crawford (2006) identifies a Puritanism emerging in the post-sixties culture that railed against the deleterious effects of, among other things, excess consumerism. Noting that an austere lifestyle would be out of kilter with a political economy where spending is essential for economic growth, Crawford demonstrates how during the 1970s this movement turned to the consumption of 'healthism' – where a preoccupation with self-help, personal responsibility and individual accountability for health and well-being emerged as a meaningful social practice – and in so doing, created a market economy ripe for private and corporate investment.

To better understand the culture of prudence that now underpins the anti-excess movement in public-health nutrition, the recent work of Raymond Tallis (2008) will be elaborated upon. Tallis' discussion of hunger provides a useful background to the current problems with the culture of excess and our (Western) disposition to frugality.

Tallis and hunger

In his book, titled *Hunger*, Tallis points out some obvious, though little considered, facts. First, unlike almost any other subjective experience, it is hunger that unites humans: we are all likely to have endured and been discomforted by it at some stage. Indeed, Tallis argues that the human body itself is attuned to address and deal with hunger, through a range of short-circuiting biochemical and physiological pathways to salvage necessary nutrients and other substrates in times of need. However, biology notwithstanding, it is the emergence of a sentience – the feeling or emotion created by hunger – that is also enduring and is culturally important. In many cases, hunger is not something that needs to be feared, but, rather, something to be conquered and even accommodated. In other words, with hunger can come an appreciation of what are basic human experiences – experiences that are corrupted in a world where access to what we *want* vastly outweighs what we actually *need*. There is a special feeling about self-denial, especially when putting the needs of others ahead of one's own. The displacement or delaying of immediate pleasure with a stint of hunger is a sober reminder of our basic needs. That is, hunger is something that can be seen as useful, educative, inventive and even creative. So, while it would be foolish to wish more outright hunger on a world where there are many who are already deprived of even the most basic life-supporting elements – food, shelter and even love – in judicious and targeted amounts, hunger can be a positive experience, especially if seen more as an antidote to the great Western god: economic growth. This is especially poignant if, as Eckersley (2006) reminds us, more affluence does not always produce more happiness and material wealth is not always the road to pleasure and contentment.

The engagement with hunger has consequences for pleasure, for it addresses at least two types of pleasure experiences that have been examined elsewhere (Coveney and Bunton 2003; see also Bunton, this volume). That is to say, hunger may be part of the experience of a disciplined pleasure: pleasure that has been rationalized, and even rationed. Disciplined pleasure stands in contrast to pleasure that is derived from showy, vulgar and even risky behaviour, where immediate gratification takes priority over rationalized, reasoned pleasure and satisfaction. In other words, it is a pleasure that has to be earned. Hunger is also integral to ascetic pleasure that arises from the acknowledgment of total control over bodily urges. For many, this is a pleasure derived from a total conquering and domination of the body and can be found in the testimonies of people who have self-starved with conditions like anorexia nervosa. While not promoting disordered eating, public health does favour restraint in the face of excess. In the rest of this chapter, we examine the manifestations of responses to excess. We will draw on the response to the obesity problem, which is currently at the top of the agenda for many jurisdictions.

The crisis of excess embodied in the 'o' problem

The issue of population size and weight has engaged numerous groups, organizations and institutes whose whole reason for existence is obesity prevention and management (International Society for the Study of Obesity 2006). The obesity problem – now regarded to be an 'epidemic' – is seen to be spreading across the globe, affecting developing as well as developed countries. The problem is also seen to sweep across populations within countries, reaching down into almost every age group and across genders and social categories. The notion of obesity portrayed as an epidemic gives a powerful impetus to it as a problem, even a series of crises (Coveney 2008; see also Mair's and LeBesco's chapters in this volume). The first of these is a medical crisis, where a correlation between overweight and obesity and a number of health problems has been asserted.[1] These problems are said to range from diseases like diabetes, heart diseases, stroke and some cancers, to others less common, such as polycystic ovarian disease and infertility in women (Caterson 2003; see McNaughton, this volume). Further, the cost of treating obesity-related diseases is regarded to be of concern. The sheer pressure on the health and medical system is represented as a crisis and is now almost daily news (Medical News 2008). Obesity is also portrayed as affecting children's health. It is not uncommon to learn that children today may not live as long as current adult generations because they are likely to be visited by diet-related diseases at an earlier age (Cole 2006).

A second crisis said to be precipitated by the obesity epidemic is one of social dimensions. The groups that are most vulnerable are those of low income and low socio-economic status (Friel and Broom 2007). Thus, the obesity crisis is said to further widen the gap between those with least and those with most. The reasons why less-well-off groups are believed to be more likely to be overweight or obese are complex. Whatever the causes, however, the impact of obesity on the widening gap is seen as a cause for alarm in public health.

The next crisis precipitated by obesity is one of socio-cultural dimensions. From a time when girth was a sign of affluence and higher social status, body size is now inversely related to prestige and social cachet. Indeed, the stigmatization of obesity has become an area of concern as it creates social distinctions and even barriers to social standing. Thus it has become evident that people with larger body sizes are discriminated against in employment and social mobility (Sobal 1999). Moral judgements are exercised against people with larger body sizes while the media portrays overweight people as out of control and even reckless (Saguy and Almeling 2008; LeBesco, this volume).

A final crisis that has emanated from rising levels of obesity is directed to environmental concerns. Foods that are risk factors for obesity and so-called diseases of lifestyle are themselves regarded to be greater generators of greenhouse gas emissions.[2] So, for example, agriculture is believed to contribute about 20 per cent of all greenhouse-gas emissions: the production of meat, meat products and dairy foods contribute the greatest category of agricultural products to greenhouse gases through the production of CO_2 and other highly potent greenhouse gases like nitrous oxide and methane (McMichael *et al.* 2007). Thus, it is not hard to imagine how both overweight and obesity and global warming may be regarded as emanating from similar causes. Indeed, overweight and obese people have been blamed for causing climate change (Jackson 2009).

The term 'obesogenic environment' (Swinburn *et al.* 1999) is used widely in public health. However, the term glosses a number of important concerns that underlie both the considered origins of overweight and obesity and of environmental destruction, i.e. that of a consuming culture. As put by Dixon *et al.* (2006), an obesogenic environment is part of a wider so-called 'consumptogenic' environment, one that promotes the over-consumption of a range of goods and services to the detriment of population health. Consumptogenic environments are said to encourage so-called 'dangerous consumptions', many of which have health consequences, like excess eating, drinking and drug taking etc., or social consequences, like addictions to gambling or pornography. Consumptogenic environments are embedded in specific political economies that justify continued economic growth as essential to political and social stability. Indeed, so everyday and unremarkable is the environment of consumption, that any attempt to deal with the purported consequences, such as addressing overweight and obesity, becomes in itself an exercise in antisocial behaviour and possible ostracism (see Dixon and Broom 2007).

An anticonsumptogenic environment is a perfect motif to rally around for the improvement of human and environmental health. Addressing a widespread public yearning to consume is, however, no easy task and inevitably public health is forced to problematize acts of consumption that are believed to be risky or harmful to health. At the heart of anxiety about a consumptogenic disposition is the concern about unregulated appetites and pleasures. A perpetration of 'want it–have it' culture has, in the eyes of many, been at the foundation of many recent and ancient social problems.

Anti-hubris living

The abhorrence of hubris and unregulated pleasure goes deep into Western culture. Foucault shows how in Ancient Greece a regulation of pleasure – especially that of the natural appetite – was part of the elaboration of an individual's life, and the pursuit of selfhood became a work of art in relation to a moral experience (Foucault 1996: 451). The transmutation of this culture into early Christianity saw the expunging of pleasure as moderation, and a rise in ascetic practices that were regarded as liberating.

One important ascetic practice in early Christianity was fasting and hunger endurance. According to Tremolieres (1975: 74), 'The spiritual act of fasting in archaic societies manifests itself in a series of mystical practices – the confession of sins, prayer, reclusion, humiliation, contrition, isolation which were always associated with abstinence from food.' Within early Christian practices there were tensions between indulgence and asceticism. The tensions were to do with the 'leasing of emotions and passions, and a taming of the flesh' (Curran 1989: 105). In other words, there was a conflict around training one's natural tendencies; food and eating represented this problem for early Christians in a number of ways. First, as outlined by the early Christian John Cassian (AD 360–435), greed – especially with food and drink – is associated with fornication on the basis of the following. Both food and fornication are products of a 'natural' appetite; they are, therefore, very hard to cure. Also, an overindulgence in food and drink fuels the urge to commit fornication (Foucault 1990: 228). Thus food and drink were prime targets for ascetic practices.

Second, food was a problem for early Christians because of its externality (Curran 1989: 104). In early Christian movements, contact with the 'outside' world was considered to be a form of pollution, especially through polluting one's thoughts and ideas. A ready parallel was drawn between pollution of thoughts from outside and of food, a substance also taken in from outside. The problem of self-pollution, through impure thoughts and erotic dreams, or through deeds such as excessive eating, became a major concern (Foucault 1990: 236).

A third reason for the problem of food for the early Christian is explained in terms of Augustinian theology. This decreed that there was a limited amount of energy available and life was a struggle whereby the body and the soul could either cooperate or compete for this energy. Body and soul are therefore antithetical forces, where 'passions entice the soul from the things of the spirit and focus attention on the things of the senses' (Hinnebusch 1965: 133). Fasting and celibacy redirected the power from the body to the soul, nourished the spirit, and strengthened the individual in the life of grace.

For early Christians, strict conduct that limited the pleasures of eating provided solutions to the ethical concern that food represented. While, for the early Greeks, self-restraint through moderation gave one a freedom from enslavement to oneself, Christians saw freedom to be related to one's ability to free oneself from one's 'flesh', thereby allowing a passage to purification and perfection (Curran 1989: 104). These freedoms have very different kinds of purposes or outcomes. For the Greeks, the goal was a freedom to lead a beautiful existence in *this life*. For early Christians, it was freedom to live a beautiful existence for eternity in the *afterlife*. For early Greeks, excess or hubris was not punishable in any sense; it was instead considered to be ugly, but rectifiable through exercises that restored one's mastery over oneself (Foucault 1986: 349), thereby restoring pleasure to its proper place. By contrast, an excess of pleasure for Christians was considered to be a mortal sin requiring penance and punishment. Pleasure had to be denied. This was the route to the perfect existence.

At the heart of many of these early Christian practices was the central role of hunger, both literally and metaphorically speaking. The fall in the Garden of Eden was the origin of the sullied nature of human spirituality, which required forevermore a journey of redemption. This thinking was embedded in the puritanical belief system perpetrated especially by Calvin and other reformation pioneers. It emphasized the hunger humans have for the Almighty's majesty, power and glory (Manschereck 1985: 188).

The yearning that is part of the human condition is explored by Tallis, who writes that hungering for things we do not yet enjoy is an abiding force in human cultures, and is at the heart of many desires and pleasures. The management of this force is found in self-denial, which is practised in many religious contexts. We have already mentioned Christianity, but other forms of religion also routinely practise denying the body food. Most obvious is the fast of Ramadan in Islam, where the purpose of hunger is to remind the self and the body of what it is like to go without. Of course, during Ramadan, Muslims deny themselves more than food: sex and other pleasures are also forgone to inculcate modesty, temperance and spirituality.

Temperance in relation to pleasure is itself at home in the field of public health. Many modern-day public-health principles have their roots in the nineteenth-century movements to curtail excess and abuse of the body. It is commonly held that these moral crusades were more about salvation of the spirit than health of the body. However, the material body was of core concern and the theology and reverence of the body as the temple of God may be found in some of the reformist Protestant religions. For early reformers like Martin Luther and John Calvin, the embodiment of Christ in men and women meant that His temple, the body, was to be kept clean and pure (Braaten 1976: 16–17). Such beliefs drew explicitly on Pauline doctrine (where the body is the temple of the Holy Spirit) and thus a 'theology of hygiene' emanates from ascetic Protestant movements in which self-purification of the soul through Christian practices runs parallel to self-purification of the body through strict dietary practices.

The reversion to hunger – if not the experience, then certainly the principle – is at the heart of anti-consumptogenic movements. To deny oneself and one's body the pleasures of consumerism in the name of sustainability of one's health and environment is itself a form of pleasure: the pleasure of virtue. Thus the parsimony encouraged by anti-consumptogenic movements speaks to a hunger that is to be endured and conquered. However, far from the use of this hunger as a reminder of what is possible in a world without wants and needs, the hunger itself becomes the endpoint. We next explore the ways in which this position is captured in a number of projects that are believed to counter consumptogenesis.

Cooking skills as life skills

The movement of anti-consumptogenesis supports a number of initiatives that have gained traction in fields like public-health nutrition. One strong imperative concerns a resurrection of the teaching of cooking skills. This imperative has been fuelled by the belief that a loss of cooking skills has created an over-reliance on pre-prepared foods, many of which may contribute to the energy-dense, nutrient-poor diets that are part of the obesity 'epidemic'. In a review of the literature, Begley and Gallegos (2010) add that another stimulus to the movement towards cooking skills arises from the observation in Australia, at least, that cooking is no longer taught in secondary schools, and that a generation of children are uneducated about the basics of cooking and food preparation. Again the connection to rising levels of obesity is made.

The rise in the availability and acceptability of convenience foods is not only seen as a product of aggressive marketing, but also the development of rising individualism, characterized by the creation of a consumer, unwilling or unable to attempt to make informed choices about the food they eat. Indeed, cooking skills are seen very much as 'life skills': fundamental to the ability to resource and provision oneself adequately. Cooking, however, is differentiated from merely assembling ingredients, without any meaningful use of the skills required to efficiently transform foods into meals or dishes. Cooking skills have reappeared on the agenda for public-health nutrition. Arguably this is partly to do with the popularity of media cooking programmes, especially those of Jamie Oliver, which may have brought the tuition of cooking out from a dowdy image of home economics. But it is also part of the anti-consumptogenic movement that attempts to reduce people's reliance on the ready-meals market, and encourages a self-sufficiency and back-to-basics that may be regarded as 'empowering'.

Food gardening

Over the past five years, there has been a growing emphasis on home or backyard food gardening. Some argue that, contrary to popular belief, this is not a response to rising food costs ,which have been seen in many developed countries. Rather, the backyard food production movement was given great prominence when, on moving into the White House, one of Michelle Obama's first actions was to dig up a large area for an urban food garden (Bunting 2009). In Australia, the importance of food gardening, especially as a way of teaching children to appreciate the provenance of food, can be seen in a national campaign initiative by celebrity chef Stephanie Alexander. The Stephanie Alexander Kitchen Garden programme is nationwide, supported by over 12.5 million dollars of public funding. According to the website (Stephanie Alexander Kitchen Garden

Foundation 2010), the aim of the Stephanie Alexander Kitchen Garden programme is:

> The creation and care of a Kitchen Garden that teaches children about the natural world, about its beauty and how to care for it, how best to use the resources we have, and an appreciation for how easy it is to bring joy and wellbeing into one's life through growing, harvesting, preparing and sharing fresh, seasonal produce.

The emphasis on the 'natural' world, and making best use of the resources we have, makes clear the intentions are to encourage an appreciation of a world with finite natural resources and the need to acquire the skills to live and eat within the means available.

Farmers' markets and 'locavore' eating

It has been estimated that in the past twenty years over 3,500 new farmers' markets have emerged in the USA, and about 450 have developed in the UK (Umberger *et al.* 2008). The hallmark of the farmers' market is said to be the opportunity for producers to market directly to consumers, thereby eliminating the 'middle-man', and at the same time reducing possible distance or 'food miles' (Lang *et al.* 2009) travelled by food from production to consumption. The notion of reducing the complexity of the food supply by cutting down on the various value-adding parts of the supply chain fits well with the pared down aims of anti-consumptogenesis views about how food should be distributed (McMichael 2007). Not only does reducing food miles between producers and consumers potentially reduce the use of fossil fuels, but it also increases the opportunity to eat food that is locally grown.

Living on low-food-mile foods has given rise to the idea of the 'locavore': someone who eats food grown and produced within a particular narrow geographic radius (for example, within 100 miles). Eating locally and seasonally has also given impetus to another food trend known as Community Supported Agriculture (CSA), where consumers develop close relationships with primary producers from whom they buy food direct. This not only reduces complexity and value-adding, but also, importantly, provides an education for urban dwellers who, it is believed, would benefit from more knowledge of the production end of the food chain. It can be seen how these alternative ways of accessing food address a number of criteria already discussed. Not only are environmental and nutritional issues addressed (low food miles, emphasis on fresh, unprocessed foods, etc.), but ideological positions are justified. This last point comes into play when, in countries like Australia, supermarkets are believed to be the drivers of the food system, especially through their influence on the kinds and qualities of foods they will stock and to which they will give shelf space. And because supermarkets take a large profit in the food-supply chain, they become inevitable targets for anti-consumptogenic initiatives.

Discussion

This chapter has argued that public health, and especially public-health nutrition, has confronted what it sees as the results of a culture of excess. Evident in the rising levels of obesity, there has been a recognition of what is termed a consumptogenic environment typified by a culture saturated with consumption to the extent that it is visible on the enlarged bodies of its inhabitants and the environmentally depleted landscapes they inhabit. A consumptogenic environment is believed to be synonymous with the materialistic lifestyles seen in late or developed capitalist economies. In response, an 'anti-consumptogenic' movement has emerged, which, at its heart, promulgates the virtues of frugality and parsimony. The manifestations of this movement can be seen in initiatives to encourage back-to-basics approaches, ranging from cooking to food self-sufficiency. The benefits of these retreats from consumptogenesis are believed to go beyond the health of individuals, and to improve the environment through measures that reduce the impact of the food supply on land degradation, climate change and other factors that are regarded to impact on the Earth's resources.

While not specifically encouraging hunger in the usual sense of the term, the ethos of these movements is very much about restraint and resistance towards factors that could be seen to promote consumptogenesis. At the forefront is the need to rein in excess, which is seen to be wasteful and indulgent. These moral sentiments would have been very familiar to earlier pioneers of nutrition and healthy eating. With roots firmly in nineteenth-century Christian ideals, people like Wilbur Atwater promoted a spiritual discourse of pecuniary eating. Spiritually, nutrition functioned in a number of ways in Atwater's work: through a rationalization of food in accordance with the 'needs of nature' unnecessary waste and gluttony was eliminated. These principles are evident in the works of early Christians. *The Rule of St Benedict,* for example, written around AD 500, note the importance of an avoidance of surfeit of any kind since 'nothing is more contrary to the Christ spirit than gluttony' (St Benedict 1966). Atwater's spiritual enterprise may be understood as an ethics encouraged by a moral imperative for an 'economy of nature'. It was an action against waste and barriers to productivity. Atwater's arguments were designed to appeal to rationality and to moral reason: eating scientifically avoided waste and saved money. Economy, in the form of nutrition, was therefore both a material blessing and a moral virtue.

As with Atwater's attempts to improve the eating habits of the poorer classes, we can see the current movement of anti-consumptogenesis as an example of Foucault's governmentality. On the one hand, there is a government of others through the development of measures, metrics and calibrations that can be regarded as normative, in that they are promoted as a way of life and can be seen as similar to Foucault's 'technologies of power'. On the other hand, through the imperative to eat carefully and with a mind to the environment, the problem of consumptogenesis is constructed as a moral issue where individuals are required to problematize their food choices, consider their actions, thoughts and desires in hopes of becoming worthy, rational, 'hungry' subjects (Foucault's 'technologies of the self'). Within this rational view of eating, the sensuous properties of food – taste, flavour and pleasure – are secondary to the nutritional and environmental considerations. Indeed, early researchers debated a rationalization of the pleasures of food. Ellen Richards, an early pioneer of home economics in America, stressed that, while flavour was obviously important to the enjoyment of food, too much over-taxed the appetite and the digestive system 'like the too frequent and violent application of the whip to the willing steed' (Richards and Elliott 1910: 59). What was needed instead was 'just enough to accomplish the purpose that is nature's economy' (1910: 59). Atwater, on the other hand, could see little place for the role of flavour or pleasure since he had proved scientifically that tasteless, even repugnant food was 'healthy and digestible' (Shapiro 1986).

While it would be a mistake to see modern-day public-health practice in the same light as nineteenth-century ascetics, there is in the anticonsumptogenic backlash a strong ethos of virtue at the expense of pleasure, and the development of particular subject positions in relation to discourses of virtue. Subjects are encouraged to take up 'ethical consumption' (Barnett *et al.* 2005) or 'conscious eating' (Bittman 2009) as a means of encouraging the ethos of hunger and restraint. These practices go beyond the 'somatic individuality' described by Novas and Rose (2000), to embrace 'eco-somaticity', where there is a merging of the health of the body with the health of the planet. By extension, we can see new forms of morality opening up that requires attention not only to life itself, but also to all life that exists on the planet.

Conclusion

Addressing the problem of excess has become a new project in public health, where having too much has become as much a risk factor as having too little. The affluence that has become part and parcel of living in most parts of the developed world has resulted in too much food, too much leisure and too much waste. The machinery that drives and supports the affluence is based on a formula that has been remarkably successful: that of a market economy fuelled by production and consumption. Central to this is an advertising and promotion industry that sit closely alongside a media industry; these are the ingredients of consumptogenesis. The public-health reaction to this hubris, which has brought ill-health to both bodies and their environment, has been the development of restraint. Within this, the role of hunger is important for it is a reminder of what are real needs and genuine necessities.

Hunger brings with it its own pleasure of endurance and fortitude. To achieve this, public health has become environmentally responsive and sensitive. Support and advocacy for self-sufficiency, whether this be in the backyard or the kitchen, is now a well-recognized part of public-health nutrition policy and practice. The position gains its own strength and momentum by standing solid in the face of the well-oiled marketing machine of commerce and consumerism that promotes the very excesses that create problems of obesity and environmental degradation. It also gathers potency by drawing on values deep in Christian and other Western belief systems that abhor waste and detest hubris. While it rehearses some of the moral positions found in nineteenth-century public-health movements, it has its own portfolio of concerns – many of which chime with the increasing interest in environmentalism – and thus is likely to grow in voice and volume. The last word goes to Tallis, whose work has underpinned the analysis used in this chapter, when he says: 'We make sense of our needs and translate them into necessities, and into hungers, in general terms: our needs are the result of an interpretation based on what is generally thought and said around us.' It is this interpretation, and its communication, that is being redefined in the new movement of hunger in public health.

Notes

1 The presentation of overweight and obesity as a public-health threat has not gone without critical opposition. Gard and Wright (2005), for example, take issue with claims that support the promotion of an 'obesity epidemic'. As well as questioning the science and ideology behind the wave of concern about increasing girth, the unintended consequences of waging a war on fat, especially for children, are highlighted.
2 'Profligate' lifestyles are also seen to lead to an increase in food waste, which has been termed the 'effluent of affluence' (Stuart 2009). So we have what are termed 'emissions in vain' (Garnett 2008), where food waste squanders the energy used in production, but also releases greenhouse gases that result from disposal.

References

Barnett, C., Cloke, P., Clarke, N. and Malpass, A. (2005) 'Consuming ethics: Articulating the subjects and spaces of ethical consumption', *Antipode*, 37(1): 23–45.

Begley, A. and Gallegos, D. (2010) 'Should cooking be a dietetic competency?', *Nutrition and Dietetics*, 67: 41–46.

Bittman, M. (2009) *Food Matters: A Guide to Conscious Eating*, Pymble: Simon and Schuster.

Braaten, C. (1976) *A Practical Theology of the Body and the Food of the Earth*, New York: Harper Row.

Bunting, M. (2009) 'Digging for victory again', *Guardian*. Online, available at: www.guardian.co.uk/commentisfree/cif-green/2009/sep/10/michelle-obama-vegetable-garden (accessed 4 July 2010).

Caterson, I. (2003) 'Overweight and obesity', in J. Mann and A.S. Truswell (eds) *Essentials of Human Nutrition*, 2nd edn, Melbourne: Oxford University Press.

Cole, A. (2006) 'UK government likely to miss its target to reduce childhood obesity', *British Medical Journal*, 332: 505.

Coveney, J. (1999) 'The science and spirituality of nutrition', *Critical Public Health*, 9: 23–37.

Coveney, J. (2008) 'Children, girth and government', *Health Sociology Review*, 17: 199–213.

Coveney, J. and Bunton, R. (2003) 'In pursuit of the study of pleasure', *Health*, 7(2): 161–179.

Crawford, R. (2006) 'Health as a meaningful social practice', *Health*, 10(4): 401–420.

Crotty, P. (1995) *Good Nutrition? Fact and Fashion in Dietary Advice*, St Leonards: Allen and Unwin.

Curran, P. (1989) *Grace Before Meals: Food Ritual and Body Discipline in Convent Culture*, Urbana and Chicago: University of Illinois Press.

Dixon, J. and Broom, D. (eds) (2007) *The 7 Deadly Sins of Obesity: How the Modern World is Making Us Fat*, Sydney: University of New South Wales Press.

Dixon, J., Banwell, C. and Hinde, S. (2006) 'Consumption and health disparities: The explanatory value of theories of social contagion and social distinction', *Dangerous Consumptions Conference*, Australian National University, Canberra.

Eckersley, R. (2006) 'Is modern Western culture a health hazard?', *International Journal of Epidemiology*, 35: 252–258.

Foucault, M. (1986) 'On the genealogy of ethics: An overview of work in progress', in P. Rabinow (ed.) *The Foucault Reader*, Harmondsworth: Penguin, pp. 340–372.

Foucault, M. (1990) 'The battle for chastity', in L. Kritzman (ed.) *Michel Foucault: Politics, Philosophy, Culture Interviews and other Writings*, New York: Routledge, pp. 227–241.

Foucault, M. (1996) *Foucault Live: Collected Interviews 1961–1984*, edited by S. Lotringer, New York: Semiotext(e).

Friel, S. and Broom, D. (2007) 'Unequal society, unequal weight', in D. Broom and J. Dixon (eds) *The 7 Deadly Sins of Obesity*, Sydney: University of New South Wales Press, pp. 148–172.

Friel, S., Dangour, A., Garnett, T., Lock, K., Chalabi, Z., Roberts, I., Butler, A., Butler, C., Waage, J., McMichael, A.J. and Haines, A. (2009) 'Public health benefits of strategies to reduce greenhouse gas emissions – food and agriculture', *Lancet*, 374(9706): 2016–2025.

Gard, M. and Wright, J. (2005) *The Obesity Epidemic: Science, Morality and Ideology*, Oxford: Routledge.

Garnett, T. (2008) *Cooking Up a Storm: Food, Greenhouse Gas Emissions and Our Changing Climate*, UK: Food Climate Research Network, University of Surrey.

Hinnebusch, W. (1965) *Dominican Spirituality: Principles and Practice*, Washington, DC: Thomist Press.

International Society for the Study of Obesity (2006) *International Obesity Task-force*. Online, available at: www.iotf.org (accessed 6 July 2010).

Jackson, B. (2009) 'Fatties cause global warming', *Sun*. Online, available at: www.thesun.co.uk/sol/homepage/news/article2387203.ece (accessed 29 March 2010).

Lang, T., Barling, D. and Caraher, M. (2009) *Food Policy: Integrating Health, Environment and Sustainability*, Oxford: Oxford University Press.

LeBesco, K. (2004) *Revolting Bodies: The Struggle to Redefine Fat Identity*, Amherst: University of Massachusetts Press.

McMichael, P. (2007) 'Global developments in the food system', in M. Lawrence and T. Worsley (eds) *Public Health Nutrition: From Principles to Practice*, Sydney: Allen and Unwin, pp. 247–264.

McMichael, T., Powles, J. and Butler, C. (2007) 'Food livestock production, energy, climate change and health', *Lancet*, 370: 1253–1263.

Manschereck, C. (1985) *A History of Christianity in the World*, New Jersey: Prentice-Hall.

Medical News (2008) 'It's official! Mega-lift ambulances confirm Australia's obesity problem', *Medical News*. Online, available at: www.news-medical.net/news/2008/02/13/35231.aspx?page=2 (accessed 25 April 2010).

National Health and Medical Research Council (2009) *Australian Guidelines to Reduce Health Risks from Drinking Alcohol*, Canberra: Commonwealth of Australia.

Novas, C. and Rose, N. (2000) 'Genetic risk and the birth of the somatic individual', *Economy and Society*, 29: 484–513.

Pollan, M. (2008) *In Defense of Food*, Camberwell, Victoria: Penguin.

Powles, J. (2001) 'Healthier progress: Historical perspectives on the social and economic determinants of health', in R. Eckersley, J. Dixon and R. Douglas (eds) *The Social Origins of Health and Wellbeing*, Melbourne: Cambridge University Press, pp. 3–24.

Richards, E.H. and Elliott, S.M. (1910) *The Chemistry of Cooking and Cleaning*, Boston: Whitcomb and Barrows.

Saguy, A. and Almeling, R. (2008) 'Fat in the fire? Science, the news media and the "obesity epidemic"', *Sociological Forum*, 23(1): 53–83.

St Benedict (1966) *The Rules of St Benedict* (translated by Cardinal Gasquet), Cooper Square, New York: Publishers Inc.

Shapiro, L. (1986) *Perfection Salad: Women and Cooking at the Turn of the Century*, New York: Farrar Straus and Giroux.

Sobal, J. (1999) 'Sociological analysis of the stigmatization of obesity', in J. Germov and L. Williams (eds) *The Social Appetite: A Sociology of Food and Nutrition*, Melbourne: Oxford University Press, pp. 383–397.

Stephanie Alexander Kitchen Garden Foundation (2010) 'About the program', *Stephanie Alexander Kitchen Garden*. Online, available at: www.kitchengarden-foundation.org.au/abouttheprogram.shtml (accessed 4 July 2010).

Stiglitz, J. (2010) *Freefall: America, Free Markets, and the Sinking of the World Economy*, New York: Norton and Co.

Stuart, T. (2009) *Waste: Uncovering the Global Food Scandal*, Camberwell, Victoria: Penguin.

Swinburn, B., Egger, G. and Raza, F. (1999) 'Dissecting the obesogenic environments: The development of an application of a framework for identifying and prioritizing environmental applications for obesity', *Preventive Medicine*, 29: 563–570.

Tallis, R. (2008) *Hunger*, Stocksfield: Acumen Press.

Tremolieres, J. (1975) 'A history of dietetics', *Progress in Food and Nutrition*, 1: 65–74.

Umberger, W., Scott, E. and Stringer, R. (2008) 'Australian consumers' concerns and preference for food policy alternatives', paper presented at American Agricultural Economics Association Annual Meeting, Orlando, Florida.

Part III

Gendered bodies, gendered policies

11 From the womb to the tomb
Obesity and maternal responsibility

Darlene McNaughton

Introduction

> An increasing body of evidence suggests that obesity does indeed beget
> obesity: children of obese parents have a stronger tendency towards
> obesity.... the vicious spiral of obesity is rapidly spiralling upwards as
> this tendency is passed from parent to child.
>
> (Reece 2008: 24)

> We must look at the womb to understand what is producing today's
> obesity.
>
> (Leibowitz, quoted in Taylor 2009: 1)

As many commentators have noted, the culture of public-health policy,
practice and research has shifted in recent decades and increasingly focuses
on the regulation of private behaviour, rather than public projects and
infrastructure (Petersen 1996, 1997; Petersen and Bunton 1997; Petersen
and Lupton 1997). During this period, obesity and overweight have
become a central focus of the politics of private regulation (Petersen and
Lupton 1997: ix). In the context of an alleged global obesity epidemic,
fatness is increasingly understood as dangerous and debilitating – an
unhealthy state of being that places the individual at much greater risk of a
growing list of ailments ranging from diabetes to cancer. Since the mid-
1990s, the central trope of most obesity discourse, public-health messaging
and media commentary is 'be alarmed': because we are getting fatter at a
disturbing rate, being overweight or obese has serious health consequences
and everyone is at risk.

Within this discourse, fatness and overnutrition have also been consistently presented as a looming threat to the health and well-being of children,
most notably in Western industrialized societies (Austin 1999; Campos
2004; Gard and Wright 2005; Campos *et al.* 2006; Murray 2008). Public-
health campaigns unfailingly emphasize the short- and long-term risks of
fatness in children, the scale of the issue, the changeable nature of behaviours purported to produce fatness and the role of parents in inflicting their

'unhealthy' habits on their innocent offspring. In some quarters, there are increasing calls for legislation to control or criminalize those who 'abuse' their children through 'over-feeding' or expose them to unhealthy dietary behaviours (see Bell *et al.* 2009; LeBesco, this volume). Although fathers and more rarely same-sex partners are implicated in these statements, gender stereotypes about responsibility for feeding children are very much at play and, invariably, these inadequate or irresponsible parents are cast as mothers and as overweight or obese.

However, the alleged threat posed by fatness or overnutrition is not simply limited to children who are 'over-fed' by their parents (read 'parent'). Concerns regarding maternal obesity during pregnancy, foetal obesity and infant feeding are becoming more commonplace in scholarly research and popular commentary. Increasingly, maternal fatness is said to inhibit conception, cause recurrent miscarriage, pose a serious threat to the development and health of the foetus and have long-term implications for the future well-being of the child. Parental responsibility also looms large in these discourses, in which women in particular are held responsible for the future (fat-free) health of their offspring from the womb to the tomb.

In this chapter it is argued that core assumptions at the heart of obesity science regarding the scale of the obesity problem, the nature of the risk and where responsibility for health should fall, have been taken up uncritically in medical arenas focused on conception, pregnancy and reproduction. This in turn is providing new and disturbing opportunities for the surveillance, regulation and disciplining of 'threatening' (fat) female bodies while at the same time perpetuating a number of taken-for-grant medico-moral assumptions about individuals and the causes of fatness.

Framing obesity as risky

As many commentators have shown, discussions of health risk also serve as part of the increasing surveillance functions of modern medicine, which shifts the medical gaze from the individual to the population at large, and encourages individuals to adopt increasing vigilance over their own bodies and behaviours (Armstrong 1995; Lupton 1995). Presenting obesity as a serious health 'threat' of epidemic proportions is, among other things, an exercise in power, disciplining and surveillance (Foucault 1994) in which 'new forms of governance are creating problematic social conditions [i.e. unsatisfactory parenting, mothering] in which the state can "reasonably" intervene' (Evans *et al.* 2008: xi). Fatness is a highly visible and deeply stigmatized physical characteristic that cannot be hidden in the same way as smoking or drinking, and this makes it open to considerable surveillance and judgement (Saguy and Riley 2005: 913), particularly in the context of a medical encounter.

Within the discourses examined here, epidemiology and biomedical research are the primary sources of expertise and knowledge regarding

obesity and are characterized by a belief in law-like mathematical regulari-
ties in the population (Hacking 1990; Lupton 1995; Gard and Wright
2005). National and international obesity statistics are consistently held up
in this literature as 'evidence' that an increasing BMI equals greater risk
from a number of diseases, when, in fact, any data correlating obesity
prevalence with disease incidence is, at best, 'an indication of a possible
link between body size and health for a population' rather than an undeniable truth (Gard and Wright 2005: 101–102). Despite the certainty
expressed in these discourses and in public-health circles that 'fat is a
killer', as many critics have shown, we do not actually know exactly how
dangerous it is to be overweight (Austin 1999; Campos 2004; Gard and
Wright 2005; Campos *et al.* 2006; Murray 2008).[1] The ideology of fatness
as unhealthy and as an entirely controllable and avoidable risk to life-long
(i.e. fat-free) health is also ubiquitous in the body of literature under examination. Here, 'healthiness' acts a metaphor for self-control, self-denial and
willpower, and as a moral discourse (Crawford 1994: 1352). Indeed, when
overeating and inactivity are constructed as avoidable, 'fat bodies are read
as evidence of both preventable illness and moral failings' (Saguy and Riley
2005: 885).

Despite the inconclusive state of the evidence on obesity and its impact
on health, public-health campaigns, media reports and the medical literature urge parents to vigilantly monitor their own and their children's weight
(see Campos 2008 for a discussion). As I have previously argued (Bell *et al.*
2009), mothers are particularly singled out in obesity discourse as responsible for the body size and weight of their offspring. In contemporary biomedical and public-health discourse, a mother's work patterns (Anderson
et al., 2003; Zhu 2007) and feeding practices (Rising and Lifshitz 2005)
have both been deemed a source of 'risk' for childhood obesity – an argument that serves to reinforce traditional gender roles and stereotypes.[2] As
Lee (2008: 468) has noted, mothering in modernity is understood as 'both
the private responsibility of individual mothers, and also a matter of public
scrutiny and intervention, with mothering practices defined as "good" or
"bad" in expert and policy discourses'. Of course, ideals about what constitutes a 'good' or 'bad' mother are deeply cultural, shaped by larger
structural forces and underwritten by a range of classist, racist and sexist
assumptions (see Ristovski-Slijepcevic's and Salmon's chapters in this
volume). They are also linked to discourses of risk, wherein a 'good'
mother resists or avoids any action or activity that might be potentially
'unhealthy' for the child (Lee 2008: 468).

Breastfeeding (doomed if you do, doomed if you don't)

While maternal feeding practices more generally have received considerable
notice in the obesity literature, breastfeeding has been a particular focus of
attention. Breastfeeding is a practice that has received substantial support

from primary-care and public-health sectors in recent decades. Given its raised status as the most appropriate way to feed one's child, it can be crucial to a woman's identity as a 'good' mother (Schmeid and Lupton 2001), and women who choose not to breastfeed, or find they are unable to do so, face considerable challenges in maintaining a positive 'maternal' identity (Lee 2008).

Coinciding with a recent national report suggesting that '90% of UK born children are being formula fed after 6 months of age' (Lee 2008: 469), research into the 'protection' breastfeeding might confer *against* obesity is becoming increasingly common, with media reports on these studies including headlines such as 'Mums encouraged to breast feed in public to fight childhood obesity' (Ely Standard 2008). However, evidence of the protective effects of breastfeeding against overweight and obesity is far from convincing. For example, one study found that:

> The prevalence of obesity was significantly lower in breastfed children, and the association persisted after adjustment for socio-economic status, birth weight, and sex. The adjusted odds ratio for obesity (BMI > 98th percentile) was 0.70 (95% CI 0.61–0.80). Our results suggest that breastfeeding is associated with a reduction in childhood obesity risk.
>
> (Armstrong and Reilly 2002: 2003)

Although results such as these are statistically weak and rather inconclusive (Beyerlein *et al.* 2008), similar surveys of women and their infants are being undertaken at a furious rate, with most concluding that overweight and obese women should be specifically targeted for breastfeeding (Buyken *et al.* 2008).[3] Yet, some researchers are arguing that 'the increased glucose and insulin levels in the breast milk of mothers with diabetes may actually increase the risk of subsequent obesity in childhood' and that 'rather than being causally related to later protection against obesity, the presence of breast-feeding may actually be a marker for other factors related to leanness' (Toschke *et al.* 2002: 765–766; see also Braegger 2003).

Many of these epidemiological studies collect data on the fat status of women through the documentation of their BMI before, during and after pregnancy, on how many women breastfeed and for how long (Armstrong and Reilly 2002; Arenz *et al.* 2004). Some of these studies suggest that overweight or obese women, notably women of colour, are not breastfeeding as much as their thin counterparts (Liu *et al.* 2010). According to one study, obese women were less likely to initiate breastfeeding and 'women who were obese before pregnancy fed for 2 weeks less than their normal-weight counterparts' (Li *et al.* 2003: 931). These results have the capacity to further stigmatize fat women, especially as they make no effort to examine *why* the participants did or did not breastfeed (e.g. returning to work, shame, lactation problems, etc.) or to explore the broader socio-economic, cultural or political contexts that might have been at play.

As Petersen and Lupton (1997) have noted, the positioning of women as producing ill-health in their children has long been a central element of public-health initiatives and biomedicine more broadly. In the future, fat post-partum women who cannot breast feed, who struggle to but find it too painful, choose not to in the first instance or are advised against it because they are diabetic are going to have to work even harder than their thin compatriots to keep their identity as a good mother secure.

A search for origins

More recently, research into the origins of obesity has extended its gaze to pregnant women, whose eating habits are suspected of influencing the weight and health of their future offspring (Catalano and Ehrenberg 2006; Wu and Suzuki 2006; Rodriguez *et al.* 2008). Underwriting this literature is a view that fat women will be fat mothers and have fat babies:

> Nutrition in the womb is central for foetal development … a mother's pre-pregnancy or early pregnancy birth weight is a likely determinate of the birth weight of her child and that infant birth weight is a likely predictor for adolescent and adult weight.
>
> (Smith *et al.* 2008: 178)

One paper, entitled *Maternal and Child Obesity: The Causal Link*, encapsulates some of the key assertions regarding maternal weight and future child health and the 'cycle of obesity' (Oken 2009). The author writes:

> High maternal weight entering pregnancy increases risk for obesity and cardiometabolic complications among offspring … higher maternal gestational weight gain is associated with higher weight and consequent risk for obesity and elevated blood pressure among children … and that while these 'associations' are partly mediated by shared genes and behaviour, the abundance of human evidence, supported by extensive … animal studies, suggests that intrauterine exposure to an obese intrauterine environment programs offspring obesity risk by influencing appetite, metabolism and activity levels.
>
> (Oken 2009: 361)

For many such commentators, the source of obesity is the womb: the intrauterine environment. For Oken (2009: 362) and others, the only way to slow the obesity epidemic and improve the lives and life expectancy of future generations is to 'interrupt this cycle of obesity' by intervening throughout a woman's reproductive life: before she conceives, while she is pregnant and in the years after she has given birth (Gunderson 2009). Although several of these same commentators acknowledge that many of the findings are contradictory, based on animal studies or too weak to show any clear relationship between maternal overweight, foetal or infant obesity and long-term health effects, most call for greater levels of intervention and surveillance of overweight women (Guillaume 1999). Alongside this research are related discussions regarding the possible existence of an 'obesity gene' which is attached to commentaries about prenatal genetic diagnosis being used for obesity testing (see LeBesco 2009 for a trenchant critique).

With striking consistency, the literature emerging from reproductive medicine begins with the premise (stated or unstated) that we are in the midst of a worldwide obesity epidemic. This, it is asserted, is resulting in more women being overweight or obese prior to, during and after pregnancy, especially women of colour, poor women and those from minority groups (see, for example, Phelan 2009). The uncritical acceptance of a childhood obesity epidemic leads many to imagine the avalanche of fat women of a reproductive age that is coming and the impact this will have on healthcare systems. Acceptance of the threat of obesity and the risks it is purported to pose operates not only as a justification for the research itself, but also as a call for urgency in the generation of knowledge and for the development of immediate and earlier interventions into women's lives (pre-pregnancy) on the part of experts. The discourse constructs itself.

Fat women produce fat (unhealthy) foetuses and infants

In fat-averse societies, pregnancy is one of the few times women (particularly middle-class women) are encouraged to eat freely ('to eat for two') and gain weight legitimately without the guilt and stigma traditionally attached to an increase in body size. Not any more. For the nature of a woman's dietary and exercise habits and the conditions these are thought to create in her womb are coming under greater scrutiny. This focus on the womb is encapsulated in the recent work of Barker and colleagues who suggest that 'a woman provides her unborn baby with a "nutritional forecast" that guides metabolic development' and that 'it is experiences before birth, primarily, that are held to have a permanent legacy' with regards to the development of obesity and overweight (Barker 2004, cited in Moore and Davies 2005: 341).

Although many of these studies commonly assert that a great deal is still not known about the causes of foetal or infant overweight or obesity, the female body is increasingly the site of new research into these questions:

> inadequate or excessive energy intake is not optimal for the developing foetus. Against a history of inconsistent results, several recent studies suggest that in Western settings the balance of macronutrients

in a woman's diet can influence newborn size. Effects appear to be modest, but this relationship may not encapsulate the full significance for health of the child, as there is emerging evidence of associations with long-term metabolic functioning that are independent of birth size.

(Moore and Davies 2005: 341)

Some commentators are less moderate in their assertions, claiming that 'paediatric obesity has reached critical proportions' and is contributing to the worldwide obesity epidemic (Lieb *et al.* 2009). Other epidemiological studies argue that 'individuals who were small at birth have an increased risk of type II diabetes and cardiovascular disease in adulthood' and overweight and obesity (Grivetti, cited in Moore and Davies 2005: 341). The internal contradictions in this research are notable.

Also significant is that, although underweight and overweight are *both* constructed as a risk for mothers and babies, it is overweight and obese mothers who currently receive the greatest focus in this literature. Although there was historically much interest in underweight mothers and underweight babies, women who are considered underweight or 'normal' weight are often excluded from contemporary studies examining the impacts of weight on mothers and offspring, which commonly focus entirely on women identified as overweight or obese in terms of their BMI (>20) (see for example Callaway *et al.* 2006). This limits the possibility of drawing a broader impression of the effects of weight and diet on foetal, infant or child health, and evidences the powerful influence of ideas regarding the threat of obesity in these research areas.

Indirect links between maternal obesity and health effects in her future offspring are also being made via a focus on gestational diabetes. It has long been recognized that some women develop non-insulin-dependent diabetes mellitus (type II) during pregnancy and that for many the condition dissipates after they give birth. However, links are now being made between gestational diabetes and obesity and type II diabetes in offspring. For example, in a commentary from the *Journal of the Australian Medical Association* entitled 'Maternal diabetes and obesity may have lifelong impact on health of offspring', we find the following:

Many obstetricians have traditionally struggled to help diabetic women maintain good blood glucose control during pregnancy. Then, once the infant was born, everyone would give a sigh of relief.... We used to think, at least the baby's out and it's safe. Well, that baby is not safe. We have set up this child for adverse health downstream – certainly in childhood, and perhaps as an adult.... It's a vicious cycle where an obese insulin-resistant woman has an obese fetus who becomes an obese neonate, who becomes an obese child, who is at greater risk to develop type 2 diabetes.... We've always assumed that if you would just get up and get a gym membership and not drive to McDonald's, you would be able to avoid these problems.... And maybe to some extent that's true, but it might also depend on your intrauterine nutrition.

(Hampton 2004: 789)

In this literature, obesity is sometimes referred to as a disease, for example: 'In addition to being a serious disease in its own right, obesity has also added fuel to a multitude of other diseases and can be socially contagious' (Fumento, cited in Saguy and Riley 2005: 892; see also Reece 2008). It is also identified as a cause of diseases like diabetes mellitus, rather than as a symptom (Gard and Wright 2005: 95). However, overweight and obesity, like thinness, are not diseases, or diagnosable illnesses (Gard and Wright 2005: 25). Framing fat as an avoidable disease and a disease-causing agent assists in characterizing fat women of child-bearing age as irresponsible and dangerous to themselves, to their offspring and to society. They are bad citizens and bad mothers.

Maternal obesity and the unproductive and deadly womb

Women of child-bearing age are also a growing object of study into the implications of overweight and obesity on conception, miscarriage, birth defects and foetal and infant development. This research has been appearing in much greater quantities in a range of academic and practitioner-oriented journals from the fields of paediatrics, obstetrics, gynaecology, fertility, reproduction and midwifery.

Maternal fatness is now a central focus in studies on conception, where it is commonly hypothesized that overweight and obesity inhibit conception, including assisted conception with IVF, and have a role to play in infertility (Norian et al. 2005; Rajasingham et al. 2009). Again, it is poor, minority, women of colour who feature most strongly statistically:

Obesity negatively affected CP [clinical pregnancy] in all races studied; however, obese Black and White women had a lower percentage of CPs. Although both Blacks and Hispanics had a higher incidence of obesity, obesity imposed the greatest negative impact on IVF CP success in Blacks compared to other races.

(Norian et al. 2005: 249)

To address this, some practitioners are calling for greater use of gastric banding to reduce a woman's weight before she tries to conceive, but the risks are considerable, given the high mortality rates associated with this procedure. Coustan (2008: 2552) notes that one study has suggested that 'gastric banding was more effective than lifestyle intervention in inducing remission of type 2 diabetes in an obese patient'. He goes on to suggest that,

Theoretically, such interventions may reduce the risk of adverse pregnancy outcomes associated with diabetes, hypertension and obesity.
However, gastric bypass carries risks including nutritional deficiencies
because of decreased nutrient intake as well as decreased fat absorption.

(2008: 2552)

Maternal obesity has also become the focus of studies into the causes of
stillbirths and in some research is being identified as a significant cause,
alongside other factors such as age and IVF, for which there are more compelling data (Lo 2008). In recent media coverage of an Australian study into
maternal obesity and stillbirths, it was reported that 'There could be an epidemic of stillbirths in Australia in the next few years if the nation's obesity
rate continues to soar and more women aged over 35 have children' (Flenady
2008). In an interview with the study's author, it was asserted that:

> 40% of the 2000 Australian stillbirths a year are preventable if a
> woman loses any excessive weight, has children earlier and gives up
> smoking.... That's 800 babies a year which could be saved if we were
> able to remove these three modifiable factors.

(Flenady 2008: n.p.)

In contrast to these alarming and alarmist claims, a meta-analysis of
studies on the topic concluded that 'maternal obesity is associated with an
increased risk of stillbirth, although the mechanisms to explain this are not
clear' (Chu *et al.* 2007: 223).

Who gets the intervention?

In the discourses on maternal obesity, fat women are scapegoated as irresponsible mothers/parents and citizens who set a poor example, and put
their food addictions and bad habits ahead of the health of their offspring
and their very capacity to reproduce society. Framing maternal obesity and
overweight as the result of risky behaviour suggests a need for intervention
– usually in the form of education and increased surveillance. It also
implies and potentially reinforces the view that fat people are stupid or
ignorant (Saguy and Riley 2005: 886). For example, Dr Xavier Pi-Sunyer,
who runs a weight-loss clinic and is on the board of Weight Watchers
(USA), writes:

> Why does the average American woman gain weight with each preg-
> nancy and end up [after] four kids, fifty pounds heavier? It's because
> nobody alerts her to the fact that this may happen and it may not be
> good for her to end up fifteen to twenty years later fifty pounds
> heavier.

(Cited in Saguy and Riley 2005: 886)

It is argued here that within these discourses on maternal and child obesity is a shared and increasing concern regarding the 'problems' and 'threats' posed by the individualized behaviours of women whose actions are constructed as dangerous to the interests of their children, families, communities and nations. In these discourses and in obesity science more broadly, an unhealthy lifestyle is evidenced by higher than average weight, which in turn is read as evidence of a lack of self-control and of personal and civic (because of public-health costs) irresponsibility (Saguy and Riley 2005: 887). These understandings are embedded in much of the discourse examined here with little or no reflection on the deeply cultural and classist assumptions that underwrite them.

As Petersen and Lupton (1997) note, the enforcement of state-imposed regulations tends to be exercised upon the most stigmatized and powerless groups. In particular, it is women of colour, single mothers and women living in poverty who are most often identified as posing the greatest risk to their offspring and targeted for intervention and surveillance – further stigmatizing those who are already marginalized and powerless (Bell *et al.* 2009). In this literature, there is little recognition of the potential harms that arise from increased state interventions into the lives of these women, let alone consideration of the structural and contextual factors that create risks to health in the first place such as poverty, racism, disenfranchisement, poor housing, etc. This neoliberal emphasis on individual responsibility is popular because it emphasizes personal control over illness rather than requiring major changes in industrial practices, in the economy or in the government (Saguy and Riley 2005: 887).[4]

Conclusion

As many commentators have shown, the true impact of fatness on health is not known and obesity science is permeated with ambiguity and contradiction (Gard and Wright 2005). In this chapter I have argued that certain assumptions regarding the inherent dangers of fatness, on conception, pregnancy, foetuses, infants and children need to be critically examined. These include but are not limited to assumptions regarding the scale of the obesity epidemic, the nature of the risk and where responsibility for health should fall. These logics are far from neutral or objective (Austin 1999; Campos 2004; Gard and Wright 2005; Campos *et al.* 2006; Murray 2008). They also affirm certain moral, neoliberal ideas and values while at the same time rendering invisible the political economy that produces ill-health in the first place (poverty, racism, classism, sexism, etc.) (Crawford 1994).

These logics and the medico-moral assumptions that underpin them underwrite the design of studies, the examination of results and in claims about the risks of exposing foetuses, infants and children to food substances and lifestyles said to have the potential to negatively affect their health in the short and long term. Furthermore, in a search for the 'origins' of obesity, researchers are moving beyond the usual 'suspect' environments of the kitchen table, corporations and genetics as the causes of fatness, and turning their gaze to the female body and the womb.

Within these discourses it is asserted and assumed that women who exert self-control and maintain a healthy weight throughout their lives are more likely to produce children of a 'normal weight' who, according to the core assumptions of obesity science, will be healthier in the long term. By contrast, those who do not discipline themselves in these ways or do so unsuccessfully are not only less capable of reproducing, but their unhealthy lifestyles, behaviours and state of being can cause the untimely death of their unborn child, or doom those that do survive to a life of overweight ill-health and a shortened life span.

Even more disturbingly, the gaze of this deeply punitive medico-moral discourse is being expanded to encompass all women of child-bearing age because of suspicions that their body weight and eating habits before pregnancy influence the future survival and health of their offspring. However, as demonstrated above, it is the bodies, lives and bedrooms of marginalized women that are singled out for even greater degrees of health/state intervention and surveillance, and are seen to pose the greatest risk to their future and current offspring.

Notes

1 It is not clear that simple dietary intake causes many cases of overweight or obesity (Gard and Wright 2005), and yet there is little awareness of these critiques in this literature. In a review of international studies, Rolland-Cachera and Bellisle (2002) found little evidence to suggest that overweight and obese children consume more calories than other children – with the exception of children experiencing the 'highest indices of obesity', where a correlation was found between body weight and the amount of protein consumed.
2 According to one highly publicized study (Zhu 2007), it is the mother's actions adopted in response to time constraints and her struggle to fulfil her dual roles as caregiver and economic provider that have partly 'caused' growing rates of childhood obesity. In light of such discourses, it is unsurprising that research suggests that women are increasingly hostile to weight gain during pregnancy and in the years immediately after giving birth (Herring *et al.* 2008; Laraia 2009).
3 This speaks to Bell's (this volume) point that thresholds for public-health intervention are socio-political phenomena and 'scientific' standards for action are particularly low when children (or foetuses) are seen to be involved.
4 See Mair, Salmon and Ristovski-Slijepcevic's chapters in this volume for similar points regarding tobacco control, FASD and nutritional discourses.

References

Anderson, P.M., Butcher, K.F. and Levine, P.B. (2003) 'Maternal employment and overweight children', *Journal of Health Economics*, 22: 477–504.
Arenz, S., Ruckerl, R., Koletzko, B. and von Kries, R. (2004) 'Breast-feeding and

childhood obesity – a systematic review', *International Journal of Obesity Related Metabolic Disorders*, 28: 1247–1256.

Armstrong, D. (1995) 'The rise of surveillance medicine', *Sociology of Health and Illness*, 17: 393–404.

Armstrong, J. and Reilly, J.J. (2002) 'Breastfeeding and lowering the risk of child-hood obesity', *Lancet*, 359: 2003–2004.

Austin, S.B. (1999) 'Fat, loathing and public health: The complicity of science in a culture of disordered eating', *Culture, Medicine and Psychiatry*, 23: 245–268.

Bell, K., McNaughton, D. and Salmon, A. (2009) 'Medicine, morality and mother-ing: Public health discourses on foetal alcohol exposure, smoking around chil-dren and childhood overnutrition', *Critical Public Health*, 2: 155–170.

Beyerlein, A., Toschke, A.M. and von Kries, R. (2008) 'Breast-feeding and child-hood obesity: Shift of the entire BMI distribution or only the upper parts?', *Obesity*, 16: 2730–2733.

Braegger, C. (2003) 'Breast milk and childhood obesity: The Czechs weigh in', *Journal of Pediatric Gastroenterology and Nutrition*, 37(2): 210–211.

Buyken, A., Karaolis-Danckert, N., Remer, T., Bolzenius, K., Landsberg, B. and Kroke, A. (2008) 'Effects of breastfeeding on trajectories of body fat and BMI throughout childhood', *Obesity*, 16: 389–395.

Callaway, L., Prins, J., Chang, A. and McIntyre, D. (2006) 'The prevalence and impact of overweight and obesity in an Australian obstetric population', *Medical Journal of Australia*, 2: 56–59.

Campos, P. (2004) *The Obesity Myth: Why Our Obsession with Weight is Haz-ardous to Our Health*, London: Penguin.

Campos, P. (2008) 'A $10,000 obesity challenge', *Rocky Mountain News*. Online, available at: www.rockymountainnews.com/news/2008/may/20/campos-a-10000-obesity-challenge (accessed 1 June 2009).

Campos, P., Saguy, A., Ernsberger, P., Oliver, E. and Gaesser, G. (2006) 'The epi-demiology of overweight and obesity: Public health crisis or moral panic?', *Inter-national Journal of Epidemiology*, 35(1): 55–60.

Catalano, P.M. and Ehrenberg, H.M. (2006) 'The short-and long-term implications of maternal obesity on the mother and her offspring', *British Journal of Obstet-rics and Gynaecology*, July: 1126–1133.

Chu, S., Kim, S., Lau, J., Schmid, C., Dietz, P., Callaghan, W. and Curtis, K. (2007) 'Maternal obesity and risk of stillbirth: A meta analysis', *American Journal of Obstetrics and Gynaecology*, 197(3): 223–228.

Coustan, D.R. (2008) 'A 40-year-old woman with diabetes contemplating preg-nancy after gastric bypass surgery', *Journal of the American Medical Association*, 4(21): 2550–2557.

Crawford, R. (1994) 'The boundaries of the self and the unhealthy other: Reflec-tions on health, culture and AIDS', *Social Science and Medicine*, 10: 1347–1365.

Ely Standard (2008) 'Mums encouraged to breast feed in public to fight childhood obesity', *Ely Standard*. Online, available at: http://childhood-obesity-expert.com/mums-encouraged-to-breast-feed-in-public-to-fight-childhood-obesity-ely-standard-2 (accessed 1 June 2009).

Evans, J., Rich, E., Davies, B. and Allwood, R. (eds) (2008) *Education, Disordered Eating and Obesity Discourse*, London: Routledge.

Flenady, V. (2008) 'Obesity, age linked to stillbirths', *Sydney Morning Herald*. Online, available at: http://smh.com.au (accessed 12 October 2008).

Foucault, M. (1994) *The Birth of the Clinic: An Archaeology of Medical Perception*, New York: Vintage Books.

Gard, M. and Wright, J. (2005) *The Obesity Epidemic: Science, Morality and Ideology*, London: Routledge.

Guillaume, M. (1999) 'Defining obesity in childhood: Current practice', *American Journal of Clinical Nutrition*, 70: 126–130.

Gunderson, E. (2009) 'Childbearing and obesity in women: Weight before, during and after pregnancy', *Obstetrics and Gynecology Clinic of North America*, 36(2): 317–332.

Hacking, I. (1990) *The Taming of Chance*, London: Cambridge University Press.

Hampton, T. (2004) 'Maternal diabetes and obesity may have lifelong impact on health of offspring', *Journal of the American Medical Association*, 7: 789–790.

Herring, S.J., Rich-Edwards, J.W., Oken, E., Rifas-Shiman, S.L., Kleinman, K.P. and Gillman, M.W. (2008) 'Association of postpartum depression with weight retention 1 year after childbirth', *Obesity*, 16(6): 1296–1301.

Laraia, B.A. (2009) 'Pregravid weight is associated with prior dietary restraint and psychosocial factors during pregnancy', *Obesity*, 3: 550–558.

LeBesco, K. (2009) 'Quest for a cause: The fat gene, the gay gene, and the new eugenics', in E. Rothblum and S. Solovay (eds) *The Fat Studies Reader*, New York: New York University Press, pp. 65–74.

Lee, E.J. (2008) 'Living with risk in the age of "intensive motherhood": Maternal identity and infant feeding', *Risk and Society*, 5: 467–477.

Li, R., Jewell, S. and Grummer-Strawn, L. (2003) 'Maternal obesity and breast-feeding practices', *American Journal of Clinical Nutrition*, 77(4): 931–936.

Lieb, D.C., Snow, R.E. and DeBoer, M.D. (2009) 'Socioeconomic factors in the development of childhood obesity and diabetes', *Clinics in Sports Medicine*, 28(3): 349–378.

Liu, J., Smith, M.G., Dobre, M.A. and Ferguson, J.E. (2010) 'Maternal obesity and breast-feeding practices among white and black women', *Obesity*, 18(1): 175–182.

Lo, W. (2008) 'Study links obesity to recurrent miscarriage', *Royal College of Obstetricians and Gynaecologists*. Online, available at: www.rcog.org.uk/news/study-links-obesity-recurrent-miscarriage (accessed 10 October 2008).

Lupton, D. (1995) *The Imperative of Health: Public Health and the Regulated Body*, United Kingdom: Sage Publications.

Moore, V.M. and Davies, M.J. (2005) 'Diet during pregnancy, neonatal outcomes and later health', *Reproduction, Fertility and Development*, 17(3): 341–348.

Murray, S. (2008) Pathologising 'fatness': Medical authority and popular culture', *Sociology of Sport Journal*, 1: 7–21.

Norian, J.M., Hurwitz, J., Jindal, S., Lieman, H., Pal, L. and Neal-Perry, G. (2005) 'A combination of obesity and black race carries the worst prognosis in IVF clinical pregnancy outcome', *Journal of the American Medical Association*, 1: 249–250.

Oken, E. (2009) 'Maternal and child obesity: The causal link', *Obstetrics and Gynaecology Clinic of North America*, 2: 361–377.

Petersen, A. (1996) 'Risk and the regulated self: The discourse of health promotion as politics of uncertainty', *Journal of Sociology*, 1: 44–57.

Petersen, A. (1997) 'Risk, governance, and the new public health', in A. Peterson and R. Bunton (eds) *Foucault, Health and Medicine*, London: Routledge, pp. 189–206.

Petersen, A. and Bunton, R. (eds) (1997) *Foucault, Health and Medicine*, London: Routledge.

Petersen, A. and Lupton, D. (1997) *The New Public Health: Health and Self in the Age of Risk*, United Kingdom: Sage.

Phelan, S.T. (2009) 'Obesity in minority women: Calories, commerce, and culture', *Obstetrics and Gynaecology Clinic of North America*, 2: 379–392.

Rajasingham, D., Seed, P.T., Briley, A.L., Shennan, A.H. and Poston, L. (2009) 'A prospective study of pregnancy outcome and biomarkers of oxidative stress in nulliparous obese women', *American Journal of Obstetrics and Gynaecology*, 2: 395–399.

Reece, E.A. (2008) 'Perspectives on obesity, pregnancy and birth outcomes in the United States: The scope of the problem', *American Journal of Obstetrics and Gynaecology*, 1: 23–27.

Rising, R. and Lifshitz, F. (2005) 'Relationship between maternal obesity and infant feeding-interactions', *Nutrition Journal*, 4(17): 1–13.

Rodriguez, A., Miettunen, J., Henricksen, T.B., Olsen, J., Obel, C., Taanila, A., Ebeling, H., Linnet, K.M., Moilanen, I. and Jarvelin, M.R. (2008) 'Maternal adiposity prior to pregnancy is associated with ADHD symptoms in offspring: Evidence from three prospective pregnancy cohorts', *International Journal of Obesity*, 32: 550–557.

Rolland-Cachera, M.F. and Bellisle, F. (2002) 'Nutrition', in W. Burniat, T. Cole, I. Lissau and E. Poskitt (eds) *Child and Adolescent Obesity: Causes and Consequences, Prevention and Management*, Cambridge: Cambridge University Press, pp. 69–86.

Saguy, A.C. and Riley, K.W. (2005) 'Weighing both sides: Morality, mortality, and framing contests over obesity', *Journal of Health Politics*, 5: 869–921.

Schmeid, V. and Lupton, D. (2001) 'Blurring the boundaries: Breastfeeding and maternal subjectivity', *Sociology of Health and Illness*, 2: 234–250.

Smith, S.A., Hulsey, T. and Goodnight, W. (2008) 'Effects of obesity on pregnancy', *Journal of Obstetric, Gynecologic and Neonatal Nursing*, 37(2): 176–184.

Taylor, P. (2009) 'Born to love fat, thanks to mom's diet', *Globe and Mail*. Online, available at: www.theglobeandmail.com/life/article722867.ece (accessed 1 June 2009).

Toschke, A.M., Vignerova, J., Lhotska, L., Osancova, K., Koletzko, B. and von Kries, R. (2002) 'Overweight and obesity in 6-to-14-year-old Czech children in 1991: Protective effect of breast-feeding', *Journal of Pediatric Gastroenterology and Nutrition*, 141: 764–769.

Wu, Q. and Suzuki, M. (2006) 'Parental obesity and overweight affect the body-fat accumulation in the offspring: The possible effect of a high-fat diet through epigenetic inheritance', *Obesity Reviews*, 7(2): 201–208.

Zhu, A. (2007) 'The effect of maternal employment on the likelihood of a child being overweight', *School of Economics Discussion Paper 17*, Sydney: University of New South Wales.

12 Responsibility for the family's health

How nutritional discourses construct the role of mothers

Svetlana Ristovski-Slijepcevic

Introduction

Although we tend to think of mothering as something that is negotiated at home between family members, how women become mothers and live mothering is greatly determined by larger structural forces. At the broadest level,

> mothering is shaped by Western ideals and the realities of late neo-liberal capitalism. Issues of racism, classism, heterosexism, ageism, and ableism are embedded within these ideals and realities and serve to generate a range of unstated 'norms' that profoundly shape the experiences of women/mothers.
>
> (Varcoe and Hartrick Doane 2008: 298)

As with most other norms (Brandt and Rozin 1997; Foucault 1972), child rearing and feeding practices have changed (and, arguably, have become more complex) over different periods in time. In the last century or so, feeding the family nutritionally acceptable foods has become an explicitly essential part of the ethics of 'good' parenthood. Particularly since the post-war era, parents have been encouraged to simultaneously treat their children as individuals and foster their independence, while ensuring that they eat nutritious foods and in the right amounts recommended (Coveney 2000).

Although not always explicitly stated, mothers are at the centre of most public-health messages that relate to parenting, feeding, the home and the family as they are seen to hold the family's health in their hands. Because a mother's food, alcohol and smoking behaviour before she becomes pregnant, while she is carrying her child and while she is breastfeeding is believed to be crucial for the health of her child, she is to abandon all 'risky' behaviours (see McNaughton, this volume). Moreover, how mothers feed their children post-infancy and breastfeeding, and what eating habits they instil in them either through food provision or role-modelling, continue to carry moral overtones. Women are, therefore, forever scrutinized for what they consume and what they feed their off-spring in relation to their role as mothers. Significantly, the scrutiny of these practices has intensified enormously over the past decade in concert with growing public-health concerns about the alleged obesity 'epidemic' (see Bell *et al.* 2009; Gard and Wright 2005).

In this chapter, I focus on the issue of food and argue that healthy-eating discourses, though on the surface seeming to act as brokers between complicated nutritional science and everyday food practices, contribute to the social construction of a particular type of mothering, one that offers potent possibilities for discrimination and stigma towards mothers who do not follow the prescribed practices. I begin by describing the paradigms of public health through which healthy-eating messages are conveyed, I then describe the social standards constructed for mothers through healthy-eating discourses and elaborate on how some mothers are seen as 'good' and others as 'bad' according to their compliance with dominant discourses. Through this exercise, I show that via the use of moralistic language about parental responsibility and control, healthy-eating discourses may actually work to augment disparities in mothering and family health.

Nutrition as a dual scientific and moral discourse

Today, norms about eating healthfully are conveyed through discourses that present nutritional science as the dominant explanation for the relationships between food, health and well-being. Developed as part of a panoply of technologies and strategies in the Enlightenment period designed to better manage populations (Foucault 1991), nutritional science has grown as part of the population sciences used to inform the regulation of human behaviours and mundane activities (Coveney 2000).

The rationales of population sciences are today common sense, and nutritional science is converted into recommendations, guidelines and guides that nutrition experts believe are practical, meet nutrient needs, promote health and minimize risk for nutrition-related chronic diseases (Health Canada 2007). Exemplifying neoliberal underpinnings (see LeBesco, this volume), these rationales are set to reach a particular goal: according to Health Canada's *Nutrition and Health: An Agenda for Action*, 'a well nourished population contributes to a healthier, more productive, population, lower health care and social costs, and better quality of life' (Health Canada 1996). To reach this goal, however, people are expected to adopt behaviours that incorporate nutritional discourses into the practicalities of everyday food practices, as in the form of diet regimes for the family (Coveney 2000; Petersen 1996).

As several commentators have noted, discourses from nutritional science play a central role in people's understandings of food, weight and health in contemporary Western societies (Coveney 2000, 2004; Lupton 1996). Such discourses focus on people's ability to self-manage and regulate the course of their health (Castel 1991; Petersen 1996) and adopt a calculating and prudent attitude towards preventing any risk of ill-health (Petersen 1997). Risk factors are treated as if they are a disease in themselves (see Mair's and LeBesco's chapters in this volume) and they provide an opportunity to invoke individual responsibility and, therefore, moral laxity in the aetiology of a disease. Given the ease with which risk can be attributed to one's lifestyle, to moralize illness that may be related to one's diet has become unproblematic (Rozin 1997).

These disciplinary practices seem to have overshadowed and marginalized perspectives about food and health that entail less stringent self-monitoring and more acceptance of the inevitable processes of illness, ageing and dying (Ristovski-Slijepcevic *et al.* 2008). As a result, nutrition-related examinations and assessments have contributed to the production of individuals who problematize their relationship with food in terms of whether they are 'good' or 'bad' eaters, citizens or mothers (Coveney 1998, 1999a, 1999b, 2000; Holmes and Gastaldo 2002). By grounding food issues in a rational and biomedical discourse, rather than an overtly religious or ascetic discourse, as was historically the case (Coveney 2000), nutrition has redefined what it means to be 'good'. 'But now, instead of effacing the pleasure of food, modern subjects [are] able to rationalize it through moral judgements based on science' (Coveney 2000: 109; see also Coveney, this volume). Nutrition can thus be seen as not only a scientific but also a moral or ethical discipline (Coveney 2000), one that has emerged through a profound relationship between science and religion (Coveney 1999b).

Healthy-eating governance is thus a form of social control exercised by social institutions that attempt to ensure that people follow the accepted rules (Crotty 1995). Such governance deems that 'the adoption of behaviours or regimes that are presumed to improve health may be easier and more successful if these behaviours and regimes are endowed with moral meaning' (Brandt and Rozin 1997: 2–3). As Brandt and Rozin (1997: 1) observe:

> We live in a time of deep interest in – if not obsession with – the problems of health and disease.... Increasingly, we are told that new knowledge gives us new opportunities to take control of our health. With this new knowledge, however, come new responsibilities and a new set of moral expectations about health and disease.

Although it can be argued that stigmatizing certain behaviours can have a positive impact on health, it needs to be recognized that emphasizing personal responsibility also produces the potential for victim-blaming (Brandt and Rozin 1997). Setting social boundaries by defining acceptable and unacceptable lifestyles may serve the interests of particular groups in society while being socially discriminatory and exclusionary of other groups without acknowledging that lifestyle is 'only partly about health and a good deal about individual and collective social position, status, and image' (Leichter 1997: 361).

Social standards created for families and mothers

The family has become an essential focus of nutrition and other health disciplines. As Foucault (1980: 174) has pointed out: 'the family is assigned a linking role between general objectives regarding the good health of the social body and individuals' desire or need for care.' The family is not only a site for collecting information about health-related activities, but also a site for reform of normal rather than diseased populations (Armstrong 1995).

Despite evidence that a number of individual and collective factors influence children's and youths' healthy-eating practices and that factors external to the family can overshadow familial influences (Taylor *et al.* 2005), parents (mothers in particular) are deemed responsible for the health of their children. Nutrition and health experts assess families by measuring and calculating respective family members' weight and physical appearance. They also examine the foods children are given to eat, including what type, how much and how often. They question whether the family eats meals together and conduct analyses of risk based on whether parents are home when their children leave for school and return home (e.g. Videon and Manning 2003). Nutrition experts encourage parents to be 'role models in helping children to develop a taste for healthy food' (Health Canada 2008: 2) as they consider family meals to 'constitute a prevalent risk factor for poor food intake' (Videon and Manning 2003: 370). While vaguely acknowledging that the environment can pose challenges to healthy eating, the challenges are considered surmountable as the following quote suggests: '[d]espite challenges to eating well, it is possible for people to adopt healthy eating practices' (Health Canada 2008: 2).

Nutrition experts also present parents with particular parenting styles that are said to influence children's consumption of healthy foods, suggesting that parenting in a certain way ensures children consume amounts of fruit and vegetables closer to the recommended guidelines (Kremers *et al.* 2003). Today, advice about how to parent with respect to food is ubiquitous. Popular media, Internet websites and self-help manuals disseminate nutritional guidelines, along with techniques for getting children interested in food and cooking (e.g. having them involved in meal planning, shopping and cooking), strategies to control unhealthy food behaviours (e.g. making rules about the consumption of 'treats', forbidding purchases of these while at the grocery store), and techniques for incorporating healthy foods without the children knowing about them (e.g. various recipes in which the questionable vegetable is unrecognizable). Nutrition thus helps construct the lives of families around food and nutrition, and as such produces a 'regime of truth' that provides rules and guidelines about eating that inform and are informed by the data collected from individuals and populations (Coveney 2000). In this way, the family is viewed as a site for the application of nutritional science, while nutritional-science discourses offer the rationalities to shape families into practising 'good' and 'healthy' ways of living.

Within these constructions of the family and food, mothers are construed as those family members who will ensure the implementation of healthier food habits. Research conducted among families with young children has highlighted that women continue to do the vast majority of household food work (Charles and Kerr 1988), with partners' lack of participation justified through men's purported 'incompetence' in food-related tasks (Beagan *et al.* 2008). Despite potential societal shifts to more egalitarian gender ideologies in modern-day couples (Kemmer 2000), the decision to have children and the practicalities of caring for children often impede this shift and solidify a gendered division of labour around food. Thus the 'potential good mother' is born. Her moral obligations for her children's health begin with her own food choices before, during and after pregnancy, breastfeeding (see McNaughton, this volume) and continue with monitoring, assessing and disciplining the food choices of her growing children later in life (Lupton 1996). These obligations to care for the health of her children in particular ways cannot be separated from the gendered assumptions inherent in food provision for the family (Bell and Valentine 1997). Providing the family with 'proper' and nutritious meals is a key responsibility of the 'good' mother (Charles and Kerr 1988).

Thus, while feeding their children can be an empowering and gratifying experience for women, it can also reinforce embedded and essentialist assumptions about gender, food work and health responsibilities in the family (Wall 2001). In addition to her role as primary food preparer, a mother must act as the regulator of healthy eating practices and the family's expert on healthy eating knowledge. In research I have been involved in,[1] many men were quick to defer healthy eating questions to their female partners, attributing the healthful eating practices of their family to them. As one father noted, '[She] does the whole home health and safety thing and I do the work and things.... She is always concerned about healthy eating, healthy lifestyle, making sure the kids are active' (see Ristovski-Slijepcevic *et al.* in press). According to another:

> You know what, I leave that [food preparation] to her, because I do realize that some of my choices really aren't healthy. Some of the times I'll go for flavour or taste, rather than health. When it comes to the younger kids, you know she's really strict on what they eat, so she's really good that way. She can't have the rest of us then she says, 'Well, you guys are doing [unhealthy things] but you know you're not going to take these ones with you.' That's her philosophy there, so ...

The interlacing of particular family-related constructions of 'good mothers', 'proper meals', 'proper families' and 'healthy eating' are at least partially the result of the normalization of particular standards for family food practices by dietary guidelines and advice. The subject positions for mothers (and the more absent positions for fathers) are constructed through both scientific and ethical discourses. On the one hand, even though mothering practices around food were present long before they became a subject to study through empirical methods, women today are re-taught to do this via scientifically based rationales (Carter 1995; Wall 2001). On the other hand, healthy eating discourses are also used to define and delimit 'what individuals *can be* in the context of food, health and family life' (Coveney 2000: 150, emphasis in original). Discourses backed via 'scientifically rigorous studies' set a moral standard where: proper families must eat together as a family; mealtimes should allow for 'table talk'; children have to be disciplined to eat properly and to have good table manners; parents should discipline themselves in their parental responsibilities (e.g. model healthy eating for their children); parents should control or minimize take-away foods that are nutritionally suspect; cooking at home shows that the parents care for their children (and those who will not cook do not care). This kind of discourse leaves parents to presuppose that those who cannot abide by these rules – those parents who do not have time to eat together with their children often, who cannot afford a nightly 'table talk', who cannot cook daily meals or do not have the opportunity to role model healthy eating – are not 'good' parents and are setting their children up for future health problems, including the 'devastating' 'disease' of obesity.

The 'good' and 'bad' mothers

Health-inequalities policy discourses often refer to individual behaviourist explanations of poor parenting and risky behaviours, calling on parents to be 'responsible for their own health and that of their children by making appropriate and informed lifestyle choices on smoking, diet and exercise' (Department of Health, in Attree 2006). Implicitly, this responsibility rests in large part on the shoulders of mothers and such discourses serve to shape their experiences and the meanings they assign to them (Varcoe and Hartrick Doane 2008). Mothers enact or aspire to enact mothering ideals, further normalizing the particular standards set for their family around healthy eating.

In many families of dominant Western background, mothers (and other family members) draw to a large extent on dietary standards normalized by current nutritional science (Coveney 2000; Ristovski-Slijepcevic *et al.* 2008). Mothers, in particular, feel it is their role to keep up with scientific knowledge as well as 'show a bit of discipline and cook a healthy meal' (Coveney 2000: 157). Part of the enacted role as a mother now is to overtly take on the responsibility of translating complicated and continually changing scientific evidence about food into strategically prepared healthful meals for the family. According to one Canadian mother I interviewed:

> We try to have at least two meatless meals a week ... because of all the research and everything I have been reading about meats ... there is a higher cancer rate and everything in North America and it's associated with red meats and high meat consumption. And also where I have girls I have been kind of worried about how much meat they have because they are associating really high protein North American diets with osteoporosis, even though [the girls] are drinking lots of milk.... I am always trying to make sure that they have enough calcium and stuff like that because they're small boned ... [and] small framed people have a tendency to have osteoporosis.
>
> (see Ristovski-Slijepcevic *et al.* in press)

The literature shows that many mothers do communicate to their children about healthy eating, monitor their food intake, use strategies to get their children involved with food – all techniques represented in healthy eating discourses as part of the role of 'good mothers' (Coveney 2000; Ristovski-Slijepcevic *et al.* in press). These practices fall in line with the standards set by current neoliberal rationalities that place responsibility for reducing health and other social risks on individuals and families rather than higher structural forces (Castel 1991; Petersen 1996). The problem, however, is that even though these are the mothers who aspire to live up to the standard that healthy-eating discourses set for them, in the midst of ever-changing nutritional evidence and parenting rules, they will never attain 'salvation'. They will always need to do more: read more about nutrition, learn more about food, nutrition and health, and cook healthier food.

Some Canadian policy statements about healthy eating claim to recognize that learning fully about and taking responsibility for healthy eating in the family can be a challenge for some women. For example:

> While most women recognize the importance of healthy eating, some find it particularly challenging to achieve. Many women *say* they have little time and energy to devote to meal planning and preparation. Another barrier to healthy eating is conflicting messages from all sources resulting in a lack of clear, reliable and relevant information.
>
> (Health Canada 2009, emphasis added)

Yet, such statements evidence a certain degree of scepticism regarding women's proclaimed inability to achieve healthy eating guidelines (witness the use of the word 'say' in the aforementioned quote, which implies a potential distinction between women's statements and 'reality'). Moreover, the response to the barriers to healthy eating is limited to the provision of guidelines and recommendations – each consisting of statements or 'basic tools' to promote healthy eating. Thus, *Canada's Guidelines for Healthy Eating* (Health Canada 2004) summarizes the principles of healthy eating in five general statements and *Canada's Food Guide to Healthy Eating* (Health Canada 2007) provides more detailed information for the daily selection of food. It is emphasized that both guidelines are based on nutrition and food-science research summarized and updated frequently in Canada's *Nutrition Recommendations – The Report of the Scientific Review Committee*, which documents the specific nutrient intake recommendations for different categories of subpopulations, including women throughout the child-bearing years and during pregnancy.

Unfortunately, what becomes obvious is that, rather than engaging with the social, cultural and material realities that make it difficult for mothers to abide by healthy-eating rules and guidelines, educational materials acknowledge these realities with tips on how to choose healthier foods in the amounts recommended for consumption – somewhat unrealistic guidance that does not take into consideration how food is negotiated, incorporated and contested in the everyday lives of families (Beagan *et al.* 2008; Charles and Kerr 1988; Eldridge and Murcott 2000; Ristovski-Slijepcevic *et al.* in press).

Ideas about 'healthy lifestyles' and the need to exert individual control over one's health are fundamentally middle-class concepts (Attree 2006; Cockerham *et al.* 1997). Control, discipline and future-oriented goals with regard to one's health take precedence as moral duty over immediate, experiential and ethical concerns (Crawford 1994). In the same way that working towards a healthy body to attain 'the mark of distinction that separates those who deserve to succeed from those who will fail' (Crawford 1994: 1354), working towards being a 'good' mother by ensuring a healthy child will be the mark of worthiness as a mother. Not working towards this (imposed) goal will make one a flawed mother.

In the limited literature that considers the socio-economic gradients in diet, it is suggested that those who are better off consume healthier diets than those less well-to-do (Power 2005). There is evidence to suggest that income affects eating both directly (via the cost of food) and indirectly (through the dispositions towards food and eating associated with particular social-class locations) (Power 2005). There are socio-economic differences in the ways that parents draw on and use healthy eating knowledge in relation to their children's health. Parents with higher incomes are more likely to use technical terms informed by contemporary nutritional discourses, such as 'nutritional value', 'nutrients', 'adequate diet', 'vitamins' and 'fibrous stuff'. Parents with lower incomes are more likely to respond to their children's outward appearance or functional capacity with terms such as 'they are growing', '[they] aren't starving' and '[s/he] looks chubbier' (Coveney 2004). These differences are often construed as a sign that low-income parents are in need of improvement, making them the targets for education about healthy eating.

Healthy-eating experts assume that education informs and emancipates those who are not aware of or do not have information about how to eat healthily (Coveney 2004). In Canada, the underlying assumption is that if people were made aware of the scientific recommendations and informed on how to implement them through the *Food Guide*, the problem of nutritional inadequacy and poor health would be resolved (Travers 1995). But, in fact, as Attree's (2005, 2006) reviews suggest, there is little evidence that low-income mothers are ignorant of healthy food choices. Most mothers are acutely aware of nutritional messages about healthy eating and want to provide healthy foods for their children, but feel constrained by their circumstances in which they lack the means and resources. They utilize various strategies to stretch food budgets (Attree 2006; Travers 1996) and shield their children from poverty. Indeed, mothers on low incomes consider self-sacrifice to be an integral aspect of 'good' mothering. Self-worth as mothers is often expressed through their ability to maintain 'mainstream' diets for their children, despite costs to their own health (Attree 2005). In times of desperately low income, these mothers often feel that they have failed in one of their primary roles:

> I just get the kids together and say, well, I'm sorry, but this has happened, I'm afraid there'll be no dinners this week. I try to supplement [sandwiches] with soup or something to make it more like a meal.... [B]ut I still feel, God, you know, *I'm not fulfilling my role as a mother properly here.*
>
> (Cohen, in Attree 2006: 31, emphasis added)

This evidence suggests that nutrition messages do not assist in making reasonable choices but instead foster a sense of inadequacy and guilt for failing to live up to nutritional standards (Travers 1995; see Salmon, this volume, for similar points in relation to FASD prevention campaigns).

Accepting different ways of mothering

In addition to low-income mothers, positioned as problematic are a wide range of women who do not belong to the white, married, educated middle-class, including adolescent (Breheny and Stephens 2007), immigrant (McLaren and Dyck 2004; Ristovski-Slijepcevic *et al.* in press) and overweight (Warin *et al.* 2008) mothers.[2] Mothers who do not embrace (and it would seem embody) mainstream nutritional guidelines and practices may be seen as avoiding responsibility and, as such, to be in need of additional monitoring and surveillance by nutrition experts.

However, studies with these groups of mothers show the complex set of meanings through which they attempt to understand, experience and present their children with food. For some mothers, to be worried about healthy eating and weight is at odds with their own understandings of the symbolic nature of food and their gendered role in caring for the family (Warin et al. 2008). For other mothers, taking away cultural foods considered to have health-giving properties (health being defined in broader terms than nutrition/nutritious food) or not preparing foods they know their children like is considered inadequate mothering. As a South Asian mother I interviewed noted, 'If we've made dahl or subjee and the kids don't want to eat it, then we make them whatever they want to eat. We don't force the kids to eat the dahl or subjee' (see Ristovski-Slijepcevic et al. in press for further discussion). While they may not employ the dominant strategies of conveying healthy-eating information or restricting children's food consumption, at the core of their practices are goals that their children will be healthy and happy.

This research suggests that there needs to be a reconsideration of current understandings of the role of mothers in food provision. Dominant discourses on mothering that medicalize and blame women's practices need to be reconceptualized to offer multiple possibilities for how women can be 'good' mothers (Ristovski-Slijepcevic et al. in press). As Warin et al. (2008: 108) point out, 'understanding different constructions of motherhood and the positive values associated with caring and nurturing through food is crucial for health promotion programmes'.

Conclusion

In a world where 'you are what you eat' and moral assessments are made based on the food people consume (and are *assumed* to consume), mothers are placed in a particularly difficult position. The social, cultural and emotional aspects of food choice are rarely reflected in official nutritional discourses, and there is little recognition of the ways that being a 'good' mother might also be tied to nurturing or pleasure through food. While the type of mothering presented in dominant nutrition discourses is difficult for most mothers to achieve, it is particularly challenging for those who are not white and/or privileged, raising questions about the potential for current public-health nutrition strategies to effect changes in current health and social inequalities in the family. Instead, dominant healthy-eating discourses may position mothers as either 'good' or in need of reform, education and intervention. These processes can also be seen as gender-essentializing, in that through positioning the health of the family as the responsibility of women, they re-affirm women's traditional role in the family (see Haines-Saah, this volume, for similar points in relation to tobacco-control strategies).

While women who are trying to make sense of their role in ensuring a healthy family may draw on dominant healthy-eating discourses, they may also be influenced by other socially and culturally relevant discourses. In this sense, healthy-eating discourses in relation to mothering need to be positioned as they fit in the context of everyday food experiences in the family, where forms of knowledge in addition to nutritional recommendations and guidelines are recognized as legitimate (Travers 1995). Experiences of mothering and the discourses that shape those experiences vary with women's diverse social contexts, intersecting along lines of ethnicity, class, religion, sexuality and ability (Varcoe and Hartrick Doane 2008). Dominant healthy-eating discourses operate to obscure and gloss over the existence of multiple and varying forms of mothering with regard to food, stigmatizing those that do not fit with normative discourses (Varcoe and Hartrick Doane 2008).

This analysis is particularly relevant to nutrition experts and practitioners. Given the power of values embedded in scientific understandings to shape women's experiences of mothering, it is essential that practitioners pay attention to the ways in which the scientific knowledge they are imparting affects parents/mothers in their everyday life. Through their failure to recognize the value of knowledge that exists outside of dominant discourses, healthy-eating discourses construct a partial, misinformed view of mothering (Travers 1995). The discipline of nutrition thus must critically reflect on its own goals about how it sees healthy-eating discourses contributing to broader sociological and philosophical questions about the nature of a good, healthy and meaningful life. Analyses of non-dominant conceptualizations of mothering may offer opportunities for appreciating the different ways of being a 'good' mother and contextualizing our current understandings of how mothering relates to the health of families. Illuminating the political, historical and cultural forces that create moral categories, discourses and practices offers 'an opportunity to shape our world with new ideals and images in the interest of compassion and justice' (Brandt and Rozin 1997).

Notes

1 This study was conducted between 2004–2006 with 144 family members from three different ethnocultural backgrounds in Halifax and Vancouver. In each family, data was collected with women, men (if present in the family) and their children aged thirteen and over through interviews, one grocery shopping trip and one family meal observation. The study attempted to understand how food, gender, culture and health intersect in the family (Beagan *et al.* 2008; Ristovski-Slijepcevic *et al.* 2008, in press) and was the basis of my doctoral dissertation research. Gwen Chapman and Brenda Beagan were the principal investigators on the project.

2 Overweight women are problematized because of the assumption that they are encouraging fatness in their children through, for example, associations between maternal body weight and per cent body fat with infant energy intakes (Bell *et al.* 2009).

References

Armstrong, D. (1995) 'The rise of surveillance medicine', *Sociology of Health and Illness*, 17: 393–404.

Attree, P. (2005) 'Low-income mothers, nutrition and health: A systematic review of qualitative evidence', *Maternal and Child Nutrition*, 1: 227–240.

Attree, P. (2006) 'A critical analysis of UK public health policies in relation to diet and nutrition in low-income households', *Maternal and Child Nutrition*, 2: 67–78.

Beagan, B.L., Chapman, G.E., DSylva, A. and Bassett, R. (2008) 'It's just easier for me to do it: Rationalizing the family division of foodwork', *Sociology*, 42(4): 653–671.

Bell, K., McNaughton, D. and Salmon, A. (2009) 'Medicine, morality and mothering: Public health discourses on foetal alcohol exposure, smoking around children and childhood overnutrition', *Critical Public Health*, 19(2): 155–170.

Bell, D. and Valentine, G. (1997) *Consuming Geographies: We Are Where We Eat*, London: Routledge.

Brandt, A.M. and Rozin, P. (1997) 'Introduction', in A.M. Brandt and P. Rozin (eds) *Morality and Health*, New York: Routledge, pp. 1–11.

Breheny, M. and Stephens, C. (2007) 'Irreconcilable differences: Health professionals' constructions of adolescence and motherhood', *Social Science and Medicine*, 64: 112–124.

Carter, P. (1995) *Feminism, Breasts and Breast-Feeding*, New York: St. Martin's.

Castel, R. (1991) 'From dangerousness to risk', in G. Burchell, C. Gordon and P. Miller (eds) *The Foucault Effect: Studies in Governmentality*, Chicago: Chicago University Press, pp. 281–289.

Charles, N. and Kerr, M. (1988) *Women, Food and Families*, Manchester: Manchester University Press.

Cockerham, W.C., Rutten, A. and Abel, T. (1997) 'Conceptualizing contemporary health lifestyles: Moving beyond Weber', *The Sociological Quarterly*, 38: 321–342.

Coveney, J. (1998) 'The government and ethics of health promotion: The importance of Michel Foucault', *Health Education Research: Theory and Practice*, 13(3): 459–468.

Coveney, J. (1999a) 'The government of the table: Nutrition expertise and the social organisation of family food habits', in P. Germov and L. Williams (eds) *A Sociology of Food and Nutrition: The Social Appetite*, Melbourne: Oxford University Press, pp. 259–275.

Coveney, J. (1999b) 'The science and spirituality of nutrition', *Critical Public Health*, 9(1): 23–37.

Coveney, J. (2000) *Food, Morals and Meaning: The Pleasure and Anxiety of Eating*, London: Routledge.

Coveney, J. (2004) 'A qualitative study exploring socio-economic differences in parental lay knowledge of food and health: Implications for public health nutrition', *Public Health Nutrition*, 8: 290–297.

Crawford, R. (1994) 'The boundaries of the self and the unhealthy other: Reflections on health, culture and AIDS', *Social Science and Medicine*, 38: 1347–1365.

Crotty, P. (1995) *Good Nutrition? Fact and Fashion in Dietary Advice*, St. Leonards: Allen and Unwin.

Eldridge, J. and Murcott, A. (2000) 'Adolescents' dietary habits and attitudes: Unpacking the "problem" of (parental) influence', *Health: An Interdisciplinary Journal for the Social Study of Health, Illness and Medicine*, 4: 25–49.

Foucault, M. (1972) *The Archaeology of Knowledge*, New York: Pantheon Books.

Foucault, M. (1980) 'Two lectures', in C. Gordon (ed.) *Power/Knowledge: Selected Interviews and Other Writings, 1972–1977*, New York: Pantheon Books, pp. 78–108.

Foucault, M. (1991) 'Governmentality', in G. Burchell, C. Gordon and P. Miller (eds) *The Foucault Effect: Studies in Governmentality With Two Lectures By and An Interview With Michel Foucault*, Chicago: University of Chicago Press, pp. 87–104.

Gard, M. and Wright, J. (2005) *The Obesity Epidemic: Science, Morality and Ideology*, London: Routledge.

Government Canada (2009) *A Healthy Pregnancy is in Your Hands*. Online, available at: www.healthycanadians.gc.ca/hp-gs/index_e.html (accessed 20 June 2009).

Health Canada (1996) *Joint Steering Committee – Nutrition for Health: An Agenda for Action*. Online, available at: www.hc-sc.gc.ca/fn-an/nutrition/pol/nutrition_health_agenda-nutrition_virage_sante_e.html (accessed 14 October 2007).

Health Canada (2004) *Canada's Guidelines to Healthy Eating*. Online, available at: www.hc-sc.gc.ca/fn-an/nutrition/pol/action_healthy_eating-action_saine_alimentation-02-eng.php#6 (accessed 14 October 2007).

Health Canada (2007) *Eating Well With Canada's Food Guide*. Online, available at: www.hc-sc.gc.ca/fn-an/food-guide-aliment/index_e.html (accessed 16 February 2007).

Health Canada (2008) *Eating Well With Canada's Food Guide: A Resource for Educators and Communicators*. Online, available at: www.hc-sc.gc.ca/fn-an/alt_formats/hpfb-dgpsa/pdf/pubs/res-educat-eng.pdf (accessed 14 April 2010).

Health Canada (2009) *Nutrition for a Healthy Pregnancy: National Guidelines for the Childbearing Years*. Online, available at: www.hc-sc.gc.ca/fn-an/nutrition/prenatal/national_guidelines_cp-lignes_directrices_nationales_pc_e.html (accessed 18 May 2009).

Holmes, D. and Gastaldo, D. (2002) 'Nursing as a means of governmentality', *Journal of Advanced Nursing*, 38: 557–565.

Kemmer, D. (2000) 'Tradition and change in domestic roles and food preparation', *Sociology*, 34: 323–333.

Kremers, S.P.J., Brug, J., de Vries, H. and Engels, R.C.M.E. (2003) 'Parenting style and adolescent fruit consumption', *Appetite*, 41: 43–50.

Leichter, H.M. (1997) 'Lifestyle correctness and the new secular morality', in A.M. Brandt and P. Rozin (eds) *Morality and Health*, New York: Routledge, pp. 359–378.

Lupton, D. (1996) *Food, the Body and the Self*, London: Sage.

McLaren, A.T. and Dyck, I. (2004) 'Mothering, human capital, and the "ideal immigrant"', *Women's Studies International Forum*, 27: 41–54.

Petersen, A.R. (1996) 'Risk and the regulated self: The discourse of health promotion as politics of uncertainty', *Australian and New Zealand Journal of Statistics*, 32: 44–57.

Petersen, A. (1997) 'The new morality: Public health and personal conduct', in C.

O'Farrell (ed.) *Foucault: The Legacy*, Kelvin Grove: Queensland University of Technology, pp. 698–706.

Power, E.M. (2005) 'Determinants of healthy eating among low income Canadians', *Canadian Journal of Public Health*, 97: S37–S42.

Ristovski-Slijepcevic, S., Chapman, G. and Beagan, B. (2008) 'Engaging with healthy eating discourse(s): Ways of knowing about food and health in three ethnocultural groups in Canada', *Appetite*, 50: 167–178.

Ristovski-Slijepcevic, S., Chapman, G. and Beagan, B. (in press) 'Being a "good mother": Dietary governmentality in the family food practices of three ethnocultural groups in Canada', *Health: An Interdisciplinary Journal*.

Rozin, P. (1997) 'Moralization', in A.M. Brandt and P. Rozin (eds) *Morality and Health*, New York: Routledge, pp. 379–401.

Taylor, J., Evers, S. and McKenna, M. (2005) 'Determinants of healthy eating among Canadian children and youth: Scoping paper', *Canadian Journal of Public Health*, 96: S22–S29.

Travers, K.D. (1995) 'Do you teach them how to budget?' Professional discourse in the construction of health inequities', in D. Mauer and J. Sobal (eds) *Eating Agendas: Food and Nutrition as Social Problems*, New York: Walter de Gruyter, pp. 213–240.

Travers, K.D. (1996) 'The social organization of nutritional inequities', *Social Science and Medicine*, 43: 543–553.

Varcoe, C. and Hartrick Doane, G. (2008) 'Mothering and women's health', in M. Morrow, O. Hankivsky and C. Varcoe (eds) *Women's Health in Canada: Critical Perspectives on Theory and Policy*, Toronto: University of Toronto Press, pp. 297–323.

Videon, T.M. and Manning, C.K. (2003) 'Influences on adolescent eating patterns: The importance of family meals', *Journal of Adolescent Health*, 32: 365–373.

Wall, G. (2001) 'Moral constructions of motherhood in breastfeeding discourse', *Gender and Society*, 15: 592–610.

Warin, M., Turner, K., Moore, V. and Davies, M. (2008) 'Bodies, mothers and identities: Rethinking obesity and the BMI', *Sociology of Health and Illness*, 30: 97–111.

13 Pretty girls don't smoke

Gender and appearance imperatives in tobacco prevention

Rebecca J. Haines-Saah

Introduction

Past smoking and health research has focused on the tobacco industry's portrayal of gender stereotypes through brand development and advertising directed towards women (Boyd *et al.* 2003; Anderson *et al.* 2005; Toll and Ling 2005). Tobacco companies have employed paradoxical strategies in print adverts – promoting the cigarette as an object of women's emancipation, but also objectifying women's bodies through sexualized imagery (Greaves 1996). Specific to adolescence, researchers have focused on gendered representations of smoking in women's magazines, with attention to how this might influence smoking by teenage girls (Gray *et al.* 1997; Amos *et al.* 1998). In the past decade there have also been historical analyses addressing changes in the cultural imagery of women smokers (Amos and Haglund 2000; Tinkler 2006), with scholars turning a critical eye to portrayals of young smokers as 'bad girls' and rule-breakers (Jackson and Tinkler 2007). Over time, cultural representations of women smokers in Western contexts have undergone symbolic shifts, from sexist imagery that associates smoking with women who are bought by men (prostitution), to women who supposedly 'act like men' (lesbians); in tobacco advertising smoking has alternatively been portrayed as a tool to attract male attention (heterosexism) and as a strategy for 'being your own woman' (liberation) (Greaves 1996: 21–22; Amos and Haglund 2000). While past scholarship has highlighted the gendered imagery of smoking promoted by the tobacco industry and popular culture, there has been less attention given to representations of femininity seen within anti-tobacco messaging.[1]

Given this context, the purposes of this chapter are two-fold: to critically examine images of women and girls from anti-tobacco campaigns, and to illustrate how young women reproduce – and sometimes challenge – a gendered imperative of appearance over health in their narratives and photographs about smoking. In considering the gendered implications of prevention campaigns directed towards young women and girls, it is suggested that tobacco-control campaigns constitute a case *par excellence* of what Bourdieu (2001: 64) terms symbolic violence, by locating women's bodies as the 'doubly determined' body-for-others. To illustrate how anti-tobacco messaging has relied on visual representations of smoking as an unfeminine and 'ugly-making' practice, this chapter unpacks three gendered cultural archetypes of women smokers seen in contemporary prevention imagery. In conclusion, suggestions for more 'gender-appropriate' tobacco prevention are presented.

Theoretical positioning

To contextualize Bourdieu's theory of gender, it is necessary to start from his conceptualization of habitus. Habitus entails dispositions, preferences and tastes that are active and embodied schemes of classification, brought to life by people's ways of viewing, being and living in the world (i.e. acquired through practice) (Bourdieu 1990). In arguing for the social embeddedness of practice, Bourdieu posited that habitus operates to shape power dynamics within the context of relatively autonomous fields of practice (Williams 1995). In his only substantive work on gender, Bourdieu (2001) articulated a view of gender domination as unconsciously reproduced within both institutionalized and informal social fields. As with other dispositions of the habitus, gender is an embodied difference that shapes subjective meanings, and structures the forms of practice possible for women and men. As a pervasive and yet imperceptible social force, gendered symbolic violence leads women to the 'paradoxical submission' to, or misrecognition of, their domination. Hence it is through making arbitrary distinctions appear 'natural' and universal that gender domination endures. However, in Bourdieu's model of gender, women are complicit in the exercise of male power, as they are thought to internalize and reproduce a gendered social order.[2]

Particularly relevant to the present analysis is Bourdieu's view that symbolic violence is a relation of domination present in all social interactions, one that shapes subjectivities and bodies from the 'inside out'. In Bourdieu's (2001) theory, women's bodies are not solely their own, but are doubly determined bodies for others 'constantly exposed to the gaze and discourse of others' (2001: 63). In this view, one's sense of body image or self-esteem is inseparable from the structural conditions of gender relations. Bourdieu argues that women are subject to an 'unremitting discipline of femininity' (2001: 27) which dictates appropriate ways of dressing, conducting and holding the body, as well as feminine decorum in public spaces. The physical manifestation of gender is visible in what Bourdieu calls bodily hexis, or the gestures, stances, gait and comportment thought to be natural and socially appropriate for women and men. Bourdieu (1986) also acknowledged that persons are born with, or acquire, symbolic physical or bodily capital (i.e. beauty, strength) that translates into social advantage.

Aligned with previous critiques that habitus implies an overly-determined, socialized subjectivity (Jenkins 1992; Williams 1995), Bourdieu has been challenged for his premise that women are complicit 'victims' who unconsciously reproduce structures of gender domination (Wallace 2003). While a Bourdieusian approach to gender might have some limitations, it can be useful for illustrating how women's bodies are differently valued, and why young women might not directly challenge cultural archetypes embedded within anti-tobacco messaging.

The study

Carried out in Toronto, Canada, the 'Smoke, In My Eyes Project' (SIME) consisted of narrative and photographic research with twenty-five young women smokers between the ages of sixteen to nineteen. The project employed several strategies to understand how gender and smoking were seen by participants. Each young woman participated in a narrative interview where connections between smoking, appearance and identity were discussed. Young women were asked to describe images of women's tobacco use from media and popular culture that resonated with them, as well as recalling representations of women smokers from anti-tobacco campaigns. Participants were then provided with digital cameras and asked to reflect on smoking in relation to 'being a girl' using a photo captioning method similar to photovoice (Wang and Burris 1997). Following the photography exercise, a focus group was convened where participants discussed themes seen across the collection of images. The aim was to provide several opportunities for young women to reflect on, and be reflexive about, gender and smoking practices.

While very few were explicit about gender domination, participants' narrative and photographic findings referenced several 'cultural archetypes' about women smokers. Informed by Bourdieu, a cultural archetype can be described as the product of the habitus: a constellation of gender distinctions and representations that structure appropriate feminine behaviour (practice), appearance (bodily hexis) and social interactions (fields) regarding smoking. Organized around three dominant femininities of tobacco use, the cultural archetypes observed in the SIME study illustrate how the body-for-others and gendered symbolic violence figure prominently within tobacco control.

The 'Ugly Older Woman Smoker'

For young women, concern about the effects of smoking on physical appearance can supersede those related to health risks (Gilbert 2005: 236). When asked to recall anti-tobacco campaigns featuring women, several SIME participants mentioned television campaigns featuring older persons dying of smoking-related illness,

And, but most of the time its old people and I hate the ones like [whispering], 'I have a hole in my throat and I'm dying.' Or, 'I've never smoked in my life but I'm dying of lung cancer.' It's just, you know, I'm a kid that that's not a problem.

(Danika, 17)

Like Danika, eighteen-year-old Lindsay explained that, 'when you're like, the old people telling you like in the ads not to smoke [and saying], "I have cancer", those aren't really relative.' Participants also claimed to be ambivalent regarding the imagery of organs damaged by smoking-related disease (see also Dennis, this volume), as seen on mandatory warning labels on Canadian cigarette packaging:

Every time when I buy cigarettes, and I see like, they give me a pack with the teeth on it. *'This is what your teeth will look like if you smoke.'* I'm like, can I have another pack? [laughs] 'Cause I get really scared of it. I'm like, I don't want to be ugly. And like, I don't know. I'm going to get like cancer [laughs].... Well, not right now. But, what I do is bad, but it's better than being anywhere else.

(Layla, 16)

Layla's fears about becoming 'ugly' were echoed by others, who expressed apprehension about smoking accelerating facial ageing should they continue to smoke into adulthood. The archetypal image of the 'Ugly Older Woman Smoker' represented an outcome many young women feared:

I work at a grocery store ... there's this woman that comes in and she buys cigarettes and she might be 40 years old but she easily looks like she's in her late 50s. Like she's always coughing and like, just like the skin on her face and her neck and her hands.... If she wasn't a smoker, like, she would definitely look a lot younger. So yeah, you definitely notice that but um, not so much with men, I'd say. Mostly with women.

(Brynne, 17)

Similarly, Lindsay described seeing women smokers that frequently appear 'so much older than they really are':

and I was smoking a cigarette and I'm like, 'Oh my God like that's gonna be me in like ...' This woman ... is 35 and she looks like she's 10 years older. And I was like, I just flipped the cigarette and stomped it out, and I said, 'I'm not smoking any more', you know? And then two hours later I was like, 'I want a cigarette.'

(Lindsay, 18)

Through their descriptions of encounters with older women smokers, participants portrayed tobacco use as counter to the appearance investments required to maintain a young and attractive body, one that diminishes women's bodily capital (Bourdieu 1986). Thus, even as relatively 'new' smokers, young women become invested in the dominant femininity of tobacco use, reproducing the gendered body-for-others and enacting social distinctions between women as old/young and ugly/beautiful.

Representations of the 'Ugly Older Woman Smoker' have been frequent features of North American tobacco control, as seen in a 1969 smoking prevention poster, 'Smoking is Very Glamorous' (see Figure 13.1). As part of tobacco-control 'denormalization' strategies (see McCullough, this volume), this imagery aims to reinforce smoking as socially undesirable. With the intent of disrupting cultural associations between smoking and feminine glamour – sometimes referred to as 'de-glamorization' – this imagery suggests tobacco use leads not only to poor health and physical unattractiveness, but also to social disadvantage – an allusion to the loss of both material and bodily capital for the woman who persists in smoking.

Imagery of the older woman made ugly from tobacco use is a constant thread in tobacco control. Although they could not recall them by name,

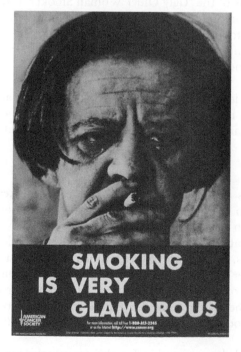

Figure 13.1 'Smoking is very glamorous' (reprinted with the permission of the American Cancer Society, Inc. from www.cancer.org. All rights reserved).

several SIME participants referenced prevention campaigns featuring women such as Barb Tarbox, an ex-fashion model and former smoker who died of lung and brain cancer in 2003. As a component of school-based tobacco education, Tarbox would sometimes shock students during presentations by suddenly removing her head covering to reveal her hair loss from chemotherapy. While undoubtedly an effective strategy with students, this exemplifies how women's bodies are positioned as living embodiment of tobacco-related disease, used as an instructive to young women that they risk losing their beauty and their health by taking up smoking. As Lupton (1995) argues, the health-promotion strategy of showcasing the ugly body in order to reaffirm the 'normal' and healthy body has contributed to a climate of surveillance where people must be continually on guard against bodily ugliness and deterioration. As a stricture of dominant femininity enacted through tobacco control, campaigns using this gendered archetype provide a symbolic warning that women will be robbed of their 'looks' if they continue to smoke, yet neglect the social conditions of women's lives that facilitate tobacco use and provide barriers to cessation.

The 'Model Non-Smoker'

In tobacco control, the antithesis of the 'Ugly Older Woman Smoker' is the young and beautiful 'Model Non-Smoker'. Although prevention generally casts tobacco use as counter to prevailing norms of femininity, in the context of popular culture, smoking is still associated with glamorous women celebrities or fashion models,

> I've always been self-conscious seeing as other people see this really short girl smoking. Like it's not as attractive you know, as a tall model elegantly like, puffing a cigarette you know, and that's one of the disadvantages I have.
>
> (Carrie, 18)

Carrie views fashion models as the epitome of the 'beautiful smoker', but feels she does not conform to this ideal. In order to tap into young women's apparent identification with fashion models and the desire to be attractive, another de-glamorization tactic is to feature models and celebrities in anti-tobacco campaigns. In contrast to the devaluation inherent in the 'Ugly Older Woman Smoker', reinstatement of women's bodily capital is suggested through images of beautiful women as non-smoker role models. An early example is the poster from the American Lung Association, 'Smoking Spoils Your Looks' (1980), featuring Brooke Shields (see Figure 13.2).

As described by the archival documentation for this image, the intent was to associate 'smoking with ugliness or absurdity and non-smoking with beauty or empowerment' (US National Library of Medicine 2003).

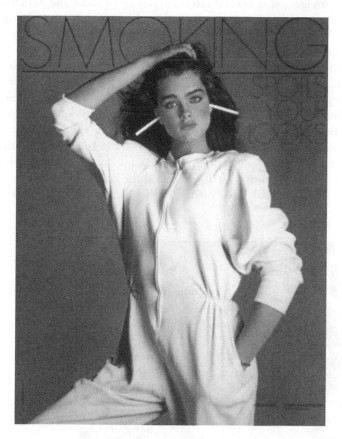

Figure 13.2 'Smoking spoils your looks' (reprinted with permission ©
2010–2011 American Lung Association. www.LungUSA.org).

Representations of smoking as anti-beauty were also seen in the 'Smoking
is Ugly' campaign, a collaboration between supermodel Christy Turlington
and the United States Centers for Disease Control's Office on Smoking and
Health in 2001.[3] Showing a serious and demure Christy Turlington, a
poster from this campaign reads: 'TOBACCO FREE. It's a beautiful thing.'
Like Turlington, American supermodel turned television personality Tyra
Banks has also used her celebrity to promote an anti-tobacco message. In
2007, the ninth season of her popular reality-television programme *America's Next Top Model* (*ANTM*) featured the show's young hopefuls participating in an anti-tobacco photo shoot, coinciding with Banks' banning all
contestants from smoking (ETOnline.com 2007). The *ANTM* images featured twelve graphic portrayals of the effects of smoking, illustrating how
tobacco makes a beautiful woman ugly and undesirable. Each image contrasts a model's glamorous pose with a cigarette in front of a dressing table

with her 'mirror image' using special effects make-up to show the devastating outcomes of smoking for appearance and health. In addition to featuring premature ageing and hair loss, other images graphically depicted stillbirth, lung cancer and tracheotomy.

A similar strategy was employed by a 2005 online campaign from Britain's National Health Service, 'Ugly Smoking'. The website featured imagery showing the progressive ageing effects of tobacco on a young and attractive model (i.e. stained teeth, wrinkled mouth). In addition to a 'Smoking and Beauty Factsheet' available for download, the site featured an anti-tobacco educational booklet styled as a fashion magazine entitled *Ugly* (see Figure 13.3). Inside, one image featured a pretty young smoker with prominent wrinkles around her mouth and the caption, 'cat's bum v. big lush lips – which would boys rather snog?' Typical of the 'nobody

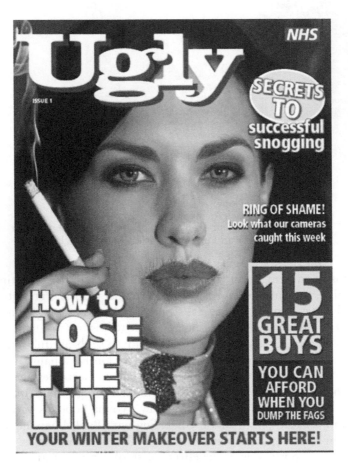

Figure 13.3 Ugly, National Health Service, UK (by Frank Herholdt. Used with the permission of Frank Herholdt and the Department of Health).

wants to kiss an ashtray' message in tobacco control (Elkind 1985), such campaigns position smoking as sexually unattractive, wherein women's bodies are valued for how they are perceived by men, and their bodily capital tied to dominant norms of beauty and (hetero)sexuality.

With the aim of changing how younger people view smoking, the problem with the 'Model Non-Smoker' imagery is that it emphasizes the preservation of bodily capital and the gendered imperative of maintaining an attractive body. Just as the tobacco industry has marketed cigarettes as a way to stay slim and attractive, imagery that promotes smoking cessation as a strategy to stay young and beautiful reinforces the idea that women's appearance is more valuable than their health (Greaves 1996). When non-smoking is equated with youthful beauty, it is possible that young women who do not identify with the so-called supermodel ideal might shun such messaging. In this way, taking up smoking could signify an unconscious divestment of feminine bodily capital and a way that young women subvert the imperative of the attractive, pleasing body-for-others (Wearing *et al.* 1994; Wearing and Wearing 2000).

The 'Contaminated Girl-Child'

A third cultural archetype at play in tobacco control is the 'Contaminated Girl-Child'. Images of the 'young and innocent' child damaged by tobacco represent another thread of visual violence within prevention campaigns, when smoking is shown to tarnish the girl-child's body. This approach was demonstrated by the Canadian campaign 'Tobacco Industry's Poster Child' (see Figure 13.4) created by British Columbia's Provincial Ministry of Health in 1998.

In an article documenting the genesis of the campaign, published in the journal *Tobacco Control* (featuring the Poster Child on the cover), the then Health Minister explained: 'It was decided to portray a young girl, about 14, because smoking among girls is increasing more rapidly in BC than among boys. *She was to be recognizably pretty*, except for the damaging effects of tobacco' (British Columbia Ministry of Health and Ministry Responsible for Seniors 1999: 128, emphasis added).

Yet, images of the 'young and pretty' girl-as-smoker hold an undeniable element of shock value for viewers, connected to the symbolic appeal of younger women as vulnerable and in need of protection (Eakin *et al.* 1996). Participants in the SIME study recalled television anti-tobacco adverts using similar tactics:

> I think it was made a few years ago, but we actually watched it in my media class. And it was of a girl who goes into the bathroom, lights up a cigarette and she's looking in the mirror and she's might be like 16, 17 and then all of a sudden as she's smoking, you see her face, like it just gets wrinkly and turns old and it's like the whole thing of like

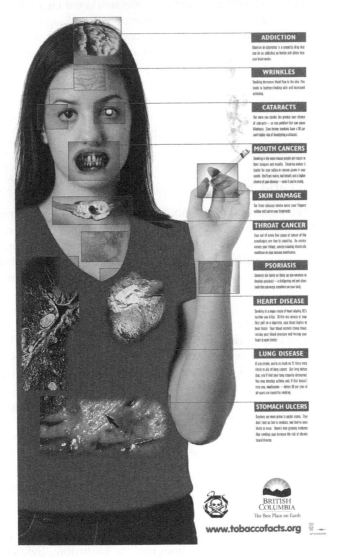

smoking progresses your ageing. Like that definitely had a bit of an impact on me because, like, something like your lungs, like you don't really see it. So a lot of people tend to ignore that. But when it's right there on your face, you're noticing things like wrinkles and things like that.

(Brynne, 17)

This strategy of showcasing future appearance-damage to children and youth has also informed new technologies in health promotion, seen in the development of computer imaging software that simulates the effects of tobacco, sun exposure and obesity on the face over time. For example, a Canadian program known as APRIL® Age Progression Software is a popular tobacco-prevention tool for children and youth used by schools and health departments across North America (Aprilage Development, Inc. 2009). Although such 'Smoking Simulation Software' demonstrates the effects of tobacco on women and men, the focus is on accelerated ageing and an unattractive facial appearance over other health consequences (see Figure 13.5).

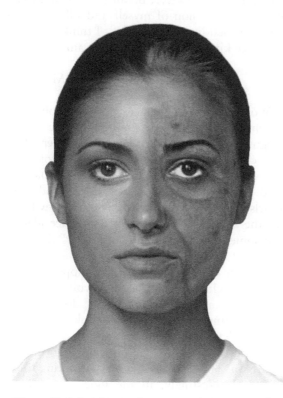

Figure 13.5 Smoking software simulation (compliments of Aprilage Development Inc. www.aprilage.com/www.age-me.com).

The theme of smoking as contradictory to an image of child-like innocence was echoed by some younger women in the study, who spoke about smoking in conflict with parental expectations about being a 'good' girl or daughter:

> I'm really close with my family and they've always been like ingraining, or putting into me all this like 'You're good. You're like the little angel.' And 'You're this good, wholesome person' ... I don't know, I always think of my family when I see myself smoking. I always think of them because they've done a good job of telling me it's bad. And I just think like if they saw me, it's like, aghh. It's like I'm a part of the family watching me, and I'm looking at me and saying 'Oh, no. The little angel girl is contaminated now.'
>
> (Mackenzie, 16)

Morgan's fear of seeing herself smoke was also tied to this archetype of the innocent girl-child:

> I have a fear of watching myself smoke.... Because I'm afraid that I'll either look like a six-year-old version of myself and I'll start crying and be like, 'What have I turned into?' [laughs] ... I think I'd like feel like I betrayed my innocence kind of thing. Like, what am I doing with my life?
>
> (Morgan, 16)

While the 'Ugly Older Woman Smoker' imagery positions tobacco use as a symbolic threat to feminine attractiveness and bodily capital for women of all ages, campaigns that use images of younger women play on cultural anxieties about the corruption of the girl-child, and evoke moral panics about the health and well-being of future generations. Similar to the possibilities for unintended consequences associated with 'Model Non-Smoker' imagery, telling girls and young women that smoking will make them ugly might reinforce the appeal of smoking as a practice identified with a 'bad girl' image and something that 'good' and 'pretty' girls do not do (Wearing et al. 1994).

Although it is significant that campaigns addressing appearance and reputation are directed almost exclusively to girls and women, it should be noted that there is also considerable symbolic violence done to men in the context of tobacco-control campaigns connecting smoking and impotence. For example, the NHS developed an anti-smoking campaign for young men in conjunction with their 'ugly smoking' campaign described above. The male counterpart was labelled 'Staying Hard', linking tobacco use and erectile dysfunction. Interestingly, in the mock magazine for young men, no male models were featured. The images and text that comprised SOFT were replete with references to stereotypical masculinity,

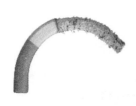

WARNING
TOBACCO USE CAN MAKE YOU IMPOTENT

Cigarettes may cause sexual impotence due to decreased blood flow to the penis. This can prevent you from having an erection.

Health Canada

Figure 13.6 'Tobacco use can make you impotent' (licensed under Health Canada Copyright).

including depictions of cars as 'boy's toys', and an image of a 'sexy nurse' accompanying a health-information piece. This text similarly reinforces gendered symbolic violence, with concerns about ageing effects marked off as 'women's problems', and young men's tobacco use linked to their capacity for sexual performance.

In an effort to combat cultural associations between 'male potency' and smoking advanced by the tobacco industry, anti-tobacco advocates have argued for increasing the profile of messaging about erectile-dysfunction risks (Davis 1998; Chapman 2006; Millet *et al.* 2006). Indeed, the visual metaphor of a bent cigarette as stand-in for a 'limp' penis has now become ubiquitous in tobacco-control campaigns (see Figure 13.7).[4] While it might be important to make male smokers aware about this health risk, messaging that focuses on young men's sex organs reinforces a gendered symbolic violence, and reifies cultural views of masculinity as linked to sexual virility (Bourdieu 2001).[5] Although there is yet to be research addressing tobacco-control imagery and young men which is analogous to the SIME study, ethnographic research with adult men has suggested that smokers disidentify with, and are resistant to, tobacco-cessation campaigns that mobilize hegemonic notions of masculinity in messaging about impotence and other male health risks (Johnson *et al.* 2009).

Challenging dominant femininities? Young women's narratives and photographs

Given the prevalence of gendered symbolic violence, it was perhaps not surprising that most SIME participants did not explicitly challenge appearance imperatives in tobacco prevention. To the contrary, some participants viewed them as appropriate and effective:

> Well, everyone is afraid of ageing right, and it just accelerates ageing so I guess and to do what I want to do you have to be young and youthful and good looking still ... especially if you're a girl, 'cause if

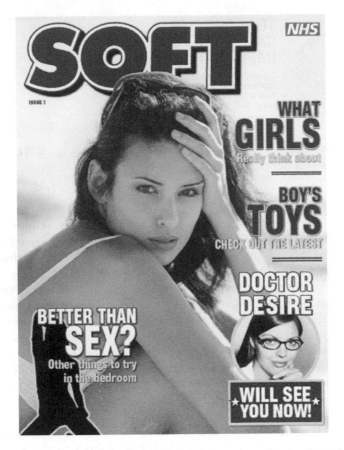

Figure 13.7 Soft, National Health Service, UK (by Frank Herholdt. Used with the permission of Frank Herholdt and the Department of Health).

you're not then you won't get stupid teenage girls idolizing you ... 'cause every girl, every woman is afraid of losing her looks right? ... 'cause that's the power she has in this world. God-given power, whatever.

(Helena, 19)

While somewhat critical of the cultural value placed on feminine beauty, Helena's statements also suggest an awareness of how women must preserve their 'god-given' bodily capital. As the gendered habitus produces a seemingly natural and unconscious reproduction of appearance concerns, young women might then misrecognize body dissatisfaction as a 'woman's problem' or an issue of self-esteem, rather than owing to the cultural imperative of the body-for-others.

However, there were some instances where young women challenged the cultural archetypes and dominant femininities at play in their encounters with formal and informal anti-tobacco discourse. For example, many young women recalled being told that 'pretty girls don't smoke' and being the recipient of similar admonishments:

> People have told me, like I have a couple of really close guy friends and they said to me like, 'Oh, you're a good looking girl but when you smoke it makes you look kind of ugly.'
>
> (Lisa, 18)

> Well, like my roommate, the one I shared an apartment with, she, all the time, she was like, 'pretty girls shouldn't smoke, that's disgusting.'
>
> (Jennifer, 18)

> Um, I was smoking outside at work and my old boss said that I shouldn't be smoking because like, he's like, 'It'll age your pretty face.' He's like, 'Do you want wrinkles?' I'm like, 'Yes.'
>
> (Layla, 16)

> It's the type of thing they say to like deter you. It's like, you just can't like call me ugly and expect me to like, give up something that I do all the time. It's like, 'go screw yourself, you're not hot either.'
>
> (Kyra, 16)

The latter two statements reflect opposition to changing one's smoking practices based on pressures from other people. As seen through Layla's flippant response to her boss and Kyra's defiant 'screw you' attitude, young women do express resistance to the imperative of being young and pretty.

Turning to the participants' photographs, there are also subtle challenges to dominant femininity in the images young women created. Beyond one-dimensional cultural archetypes, several participants depicted counter-representations of the 'everyday' girl-smoker in their images. This was seen in photos where young women adopted funny poses and mugged for the camera, where having fun with friends appeared to trump any concerns with looking attractive (see Figures 13.8 and 13.9). These images show young women posed in a relaxed or even silly manner, playing with the photography process and not overly concerned with their appearances. Rather than the de-glamorization approach employed by some tobacco-control campaigns, these decidedly anti-glamour photos provide alternate visual representations of smoking and femininity, illustrating 'what smoking looks like', beyond the constraints of feminine smoking archetypes.

In another more explicit example of critique, the so-called bad-girl smoker was also addressed in the following series (see Figure 13.10):

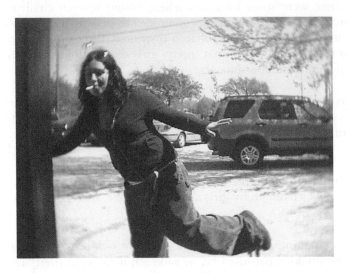

Figure 13.8 'Silly' pose – SIME study participant (photo courtesy of Rebecca Haines-Saah).

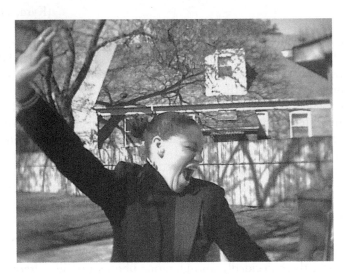

Figure 13.9 'Hype' pose – SIME study participant (photo courtesy of Rebecca Haines-Saah).

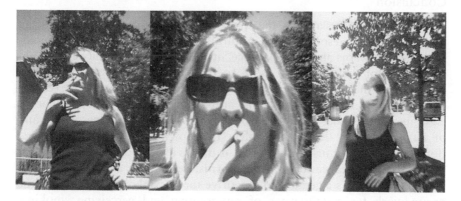

Figure 13.10 'Glam' poses – SIME study participant (photos courtesy of Rebecca Haines-Saah).

(left) – Me vamping it up for the camera: smoking is considered such an integral part of image sometimes, so I thought I'd kinda parody it by over-acting with the cigarette.

(centre) – Same bad girl smoking, but she doesn't look very cool or hot or attractive. She looks kinda dumb with the cigarette.

(right) – The bad nice-looking girl dressed all in black blowing smoke at your face. This is also a stereotype of female smokers.

The captions suggest this participant used the photography exercise to reflect on her smoking, while reproducing but yet also 'seeing her way out of' a gendered habitus of tobacco use. When this series was shown during the focus group, the other young women dismissed the participant's claim that her intent was to 'vamp it up' for the camera as a parody of women smokers. Rather, they suggested she believed that smoking made her appear attractive while she was posing for the photos, and that her captions were a disingenuous after-thought. As I have argued elsewhere (Haines *et al.* 2009), this critique draws from the adolescent imperative of intentionless 'smoking cool', which is counter to a deliberate display of feminine bodily capital. Thus while not uncomplicated, using participant-driven photography in research can allow young women to create photographs that respond to the gendered imagery of smoking. Indeed, using photo methods as a means to understand the imagery which resonates with young women might also have the potential to inform gender-specific smoking prevention campaigns that avoid unintended consequences and the reproduction of symbolic violence.

Conclusion

Through a Bourdieusian lens, the appeal of the smoking as ugly and ageing imagery is that it resonates with culturally constructed dominant femininity, where concerns about appearance, attractiveness and bodily capital are obligatory for women, much more so than they are for men. Given the emphasis on the appearance of women's bodies, smoking might be read as an unconscious strategy to make the body ugly to others, as young women enter into adolescence and must increasingly adapt to 'being perceived' and of having a body that is not solely their own, but a body-for-others. Bourdieu's stance is insightful in that it moves away from reading tobacco use as overt resistance to gendered norms, yet neither are young women helpless victims. As a gentle and repetitive force, symbolic violence lays the groundwork for certain ways of representing and perceiving smoking, reproducing a context where it is acceptable that young women's value is tied to their bodily capital and appearance.

In terms of implications for anti-tobacco messaging, there is a need to consider how an emphasis on tobacco's ageing effects contributes to symbolic violence against women smokers of all ages. Likewise, while campaigns about smoking as ugly-making are thought to resonate with youth, success might come at the cost of reinforcing an ideology of gender domination. Part of the problem in this case might be that neither those developing the content (health promotion, medicine) nor those designing the imagery (marketing, advertising) are concerned with how representations are gendered, when reaching the broadest possible audience and finding 'strong' visuals are tantamount. Finally, this form of messaging also seems counter-intuitive in that it flies in the face of the current focus within adolescent health on the promotion of 'positive' feelings about body image for young women, and the rhetoric of de-emphasizing physical appearance and challenging unobtainable weight or shape ideals as advanced by the media, fashion and beauty industries (Lacroix and Auger 2007). As much of current rhetoric in health promotion and education literature is intent on teaching girls and young women 'love' for their bodies and espouses a philosophy of 'it's what's inside that counts', with the message that 'pretty girls don't smoke' tobacco-control campaigns reinforce the imperative of women 'looking good over feeling good' (Lupton 1995), and entrench women's bodies as bodies-for-others. If one of the aims of tobacco-prevention campaigns is to 'empower' girls and young women to resist smoking, there must be increased reflexivity regarding the use of gendered imagery, so that messaging is not complicit in the reproduction of symbolic violence.

Notes

1 Greaves (1996) was the first to caution that attempts to 'de-glamorize' the imagery of women's smoking run the risk of disempowering women through campaigns that emphasize the effects of smoking on appearance as opposed to

health. Other notable exceptions include: Oaks' (2001) critique of anti-tobacco
campaigns for pregnant women, and Gilbert's (2005) work addressing young
women smokers' resistance to tobacco-prevention campaigns.
2 For feminist critiques and responses to Bourdieu, see for example: Dillabough
(2004), McLeod (2005) and Adkins and Skeggs (2005).
3 This image is available from the CDC website at: www.cdc.gov/tobacco/youth/
celebrities/christy/poster/. Turlington also developed her own anti-tobacco
website: www.smokingisugly.com.
4 Research suggests that it is one of the most memorable for smokers out of the
sixteen graphic warning labels that appear on Canadian cigarette packaging
(Hammond *et al.* 2006).
5 Bourdieu (2001: 50) also accounted for the deleterious effects of gender domination on men as 'male privilege is also a trap, and has the negative side in the permanent tension and contention, sometimes verging on the absurd, imposed on
every man to assert his manliness in all circumstances'.

References

Adkins, L. and Skeggs, B. (eds) (2005) *Feminism After Bourdieu*, Oxford: Blackwell Publishing/The Sociological Review.
Amos, A. and Haglund, M. (2000) 'From social taboo to "torch of freedom": The
marketing of cigarettes to women', *Tobacco Control*, 9: 3–8.
Amos, A., Currie, C., Gray, D. and Elton, R. (1998) 'Perceptions of fashion images
from youth magazines: Does a cigarette make a difference?', *Health Education
Research*, 13: 491–501.
Anderson, S., Glantz, S. and Ling, P.M. (2005) 'Emotions for sale: Cigarette
advertising and women's psychosocial needs', *Tobacco Control*, 14: 127–135.
Aprilage Development, Inc. (2009) *Aprilage Development, Inc.* Online, available
at: www.aprilage.com (accessed 20 April 2010).
Bourdieu, P. (1986) 'The forms of capital', in J. Richardson (ed.) *Handbook of
Theory and Research for the Sociology of Education*, New York: Greenwood
Press, pp. 241–258.
Bourdieu, P. (1990) *The Logic of Practice*, Stanford: Stanford University Press.
Bourdieu, P. (2001) *Masculine Domination*, Oxford: Polity Press.
Boyd, T., Boyd, C. and Greelee, T. (2003) 'A means to an end: Slim hopes and cig-
arette advertising', *Health Promotion Practice*, 4: 266–277.
British Columbia Ministry of Health and Ministry Responsible for Seniors (1999)
'British Columbia's "Tobacco Industry's Poster Child"': One part of a bigger
picture', *Tobacco Control*, 8: 128–131.
Chapman, S. (2006) 'Erectile dysfunction and smoking: Subverting tobacco indus-
try images of masculine potency', *Tobacco Control*, 15: 73–74.
Davis, R.M. (1998) 'The Marlboro Man needs Viagra', *Tobacco Control*, 7: 227.
Dillabough, J. (2004) 'Class, culture and the "predicaments of masculine domina-
tion": Encountering Pierre Bourdieu', *British Journal of Sociology of Education*,
25: 489–506.
Eakin, J., Robertson, A., Poland, B., Coburn, D. and Edwards, R. (1996) 'Towards
a critical social science perspective on health promotion research', *Health Promotion International*, 11: 157–165.
Elkind, A. (1985) 'The social definition of women's smoking behaviour', *Social
Science in Medicine*, 20: 1269–1278.

ETOnline.com (2007) 'America's Next Top Model's anti-smoking shoot', *ET Online*. Online, available at: www.etonline.com/news/2007/09/54371/index.html (accessed 20 April 2010).

Gilbert, E. (2005) 'Contextualizing the medical risks of cigarette smoking: Australian young women's perceptions of anti-tobacco campaigns', *Health, Risk and Society*, 7: 227–245.

Gray, D., Amos, A. and Currie, C. (1997) 'Decoding the image consumption, young people, magazines and smoking: An exploration of theoretical and methodological issues', *Health Education Research*, 12: 505–517.

Greaves, L. (1996) *Smoke Screen: Women's Smoking and Social Control*, London: Scarlet University Press.

Haines, R.J., Poland, B.D. and Johnson, J.L. (2009) 'Becoming a "real" smoker – Cultural capital in young women's accounts of substance use', *Sociology of Health and Illness*, 31: 66–80.

Hammond, D., Fong, G.T., McNeill, A., Borland, R. and Cummings, K.M. (2006) 'Effectiveness of cigarette warning labels in informing smokers about the risks of smoking: Findings from the International Tobacco Control (ITC) Four Country Survey', *Tobacco Control*, 15: iii19–iii25.

Jackson, C. and Tinkler, P. (2007) ' "Ladettes" and "modern girls": "Troublesome" young femininities', *The Sociological Review*, 55: 251–272.

Jenkins, R. (1992) *Pierre Bourdieu*, London: Routledge.

Johnson, J.L., Oliffe, J.L., Kelly, M.T., Bottorff, J.L. and LeBeau, K. (2009) 'The readings of smoking fathers: A reception analysis of tobacco cessation images', *Health Communication*, 24: 532–547.

Lacroix, C. and Auger, N. (2007) 'Beauté et tabagisme: L'utilisation des données probantes dans la prévention du tabagisme chez les jeunes', *Revue Canadienne de Santé Publique*, 98: 400–401.

Lupton, D. (1995) *The Imperative of Health: Public Health and the Regulated Body*, Beverly Hills: Sage Publications.

McLeod, J. (2005) 'Feminists re-reading Bourdieu: Old debates and new questions about gender habitus and gender change', *Theory and Research in Education*, 3: 11–30.

Millett, C., Wen, L.M., Rissel, C., Smith, A., Richters, J., Grulich, A. and de Visser, R. (2006) 'Smoking and erectile dysfunction: Findings from a representative sample of Australian men', *Tobacco Control*, 15: 136–139.

Oaks, L. (2001) *Smoking and Pregnancy: The Politics of Fetal Protection*, New Brunswick: Rutgers University Press.

Tinkler, P. (2006) *Smoke Signals: Women, Smoking and Visual Culture in Britain*, Oxford: Berg.

Toll, B.A. and Ling, P.M. (2005) 'The Virginia Slims identity crisis: An inside look at tobacco industry marketing to women', *Tobacco Control*, 14: 172–180.

United States National Library of Medicine (2003) 'Visual culture and health posters', *Anti-Tobacco Campaigns – Visuals*. Online, available at: http://profiles.nlm.nih.gov/VC/B/B/F/P (accessed 20 April 2010).

Wallace, M. (2003) 'A disconcerting brevity: Pierre Bourdieu's masculine domination', *Postmodern Culture*, 13. Online, available at: http://muse.jhu.edu/journals/postmodern_culture/v013/13.3wallace.html (accessed 20 April 2010).

Wang, C. and Burris, M. (1997) 'Photovoice: Concept, methodology, and use for participatory needs assessment', *Health Education and Behaviour*, 24: 369–387.

Wearing, B. and Wearing, S. (2000) 'Smoking as a fashion accessory in the 90's: Conspicuous consumption, identity and adolescent women's leisure choices', *Leisure Studies*, 19: 45–58.

Wearing, B., Wearing, S. and Kelly, K. (1994) 'Adolescent women, identity and smoking: Leisure experience as resistance', *Sociology of Health and Illness*, 16: 626–643.

Williams, S.J. (1995) 'Theorising class, health and lifestyles: Can Bourdieu help us?', *Sociology of Health and Illness*, 17: 577–604.

14 Aboriginal mothering, FASD prevention and the contestations of neoliberal citizenship

Amy Salmon

Introduction

Over the last twenty-five years, Aboriginal leaders, community advocates, children's and women's health specialists and Canadian government agencies have drawn increasing attention to the perceived need to undertake targeted initiatives to prevent foetal alcohol spectrum disorder (FASD) in indigenous communities. In pursuit of this goal, a range of prevention campaigns have been undertaken – generally with funding from the state – urging pregnant women to abstain from alcohol. Because both risk and protective factors for FASD are intertwined with the social conditions in which women become pregnant, give birth to and mother their children, FASD prevention campaigns targeting Aboriginal communities suggest possibilities that are both provocative and problematic for advancing movements for social justice, decolonization, and improved maternal and child health. In this chapter, I consider how gendered and racialized legacies of colonization buttress concerns for the health and well-being of indigenous children in ways that shape contemporary state-funded efforts to prevent FASD in Canada. In so doing, I examine the intersection of neoliberal economic and political trajectories of Canadian state formation with some aspects of decolonization movements to raise important questions about when, how and under what conditions colonial states support FASD prevention efforts among indigenous peoples.

Foetal alcohol spectrum disorder: What is it? Who has it? How is it prevented?

FASD is an umbrella term describing a range of conditions – including characteristic facial patterns and brain injuries resulting in cognitive impairments and developmental delays – that are precipitated by a foetus's *in utero* exposure to alcohol (Clarren and Smith 1978). There are no definitive epidemiological data documenting incidence or prevalence of FASD in Canada. US data indicate that FASD is found in between 3–6 per 1,000 live births (CDC 2002). However, data derived from some individual First

Nation communities in Canada suggest that incidence in these locales is much higher – ranging from 25 per 1,000 (Asante and Nelms-Matzke 1985) to 190 per 1,000 (Robinson *et al.* 1987). Consequently, FASD has been labelled a 'crisis situation' among Aboriginal peoples in Canada (Tait 2000, 2003; see also Van Bibber 1997). However, it is important to note that data on incidence and prevalence of FASD have only been collected to date in communities where local leaders have raised FASD as a concern. No representative population-level data are available from Canadian First Nation, Inuit or Métis communities across Canada as a whole.[1]

Because FASD has been directly linked to alcohol consumption during pregnancy, it has emerged on the public-health landscape as a rare instance of an identifiable spectrum of 'birth defects' and 'developmental disabilities' which are '100 per cent preventable' – provided pregnant women stop drinking (see Armstrong 2003). In Canada it appears that between 11–15 per cent of women consumed alcohol during their last pregnancy (Environics Research Group 2006; Poole and Dell 2005). If this is the case, alcohol use in pregnancy is much less common in Canada than in other countries. For example, a survey of non-indigenous pregnant women in Western Australia reported that 58.7 per cent consumed alcohol at some point in their pregnancy (Colvin *et al.* 2007). A 2005 UK study reported that 54 per cent of pregnant women consumed alcohol – the same proportion of pregnant women reporting having taken iron and/or vitamin supplements (Bollin *et al.* 2007). There are presently no population-level data showing the extent to which Aboriginal women in Canada drink during pregnancy, or if Aboriginal women's alcohol use varies by age, income level, education, employment status, place of residence, cultural affiliation, or any other factors that have been shown to differentiate alcohol-use patterns in other populations of non-indigenous Canadian women (Adlaf *et al.* 2005).

As women's alcohol use during pregnancy varies widely across national contexts, so too does the advice given to pregnant women about whether or how much they should drink. Because no lower limit of alcohol exposure has been established to create a threshold for absolute safety, Health Canada (1996), the US Surgeon General (2005), the Royal Australian and New Zealand College of Obstetricians and Gynaecologists (2008) and the British Medical Association (2007) have taken a cautionary approach in advising women to abstain from alcohol completely while they are pregnant. Others, such as the British Royal College of Obstetricians and Gynaecologists (2006: 1), counsel that 'it remains the case that there is no evidence of harm from low levels of alcohol consumption, defined as no more than one or two units of alcohol once or twice a week'.

What is clear is that both the incidence and prevalence of alcohol use in pregnancy seem to be changing. This is primarily due to the fact that those women whose drinking patterns were 'low risk' to begin with are now abstaining completely. However, rates of episodic high-volume and high-frequency drinking (often referred to as 'binge-drinking') among pregnant women (and non-pregnant women of child-bearing age) have remained relatively stable (Poole and Dell 2005; US Surgeon General 2005). It is these drinking patterns that are presently believed to be most closely associated with the likelihood of having a child with FASD (Floyd et al. 2007; Maier and West 2001; May et al. 2004).

The health and wealth of the nation: maternal education campaigns and the prevention of FASD

Public-health education campaigns directed towards mothers and aimed at improving infant and child health have been key features of the Canadian public-health landscape for over 100 years as a relatively inexpensive and uncontroversial means of showing that some policy attention is being paid to health inequities (Arnup 1994). It is certainly the case that informational pamphlets, posters, television and radio advertisements, and other usual suspects in the new public health's primary prevention arsenal, consume considerable state resources. However, these interventions are comparatively easier and cheaper to conduct than are systemic changes aimed at addressing the root causes of health inequities which place profound constraints on some women's efforts to ensure the well-being of their children.

Feminist and anti-racist scholarship on the social construction of mothering has highlighted the numerous ways in which women, and most particularly those further marginalized by race, class and disability, are punished through state-sponsored disciplinary regimes for failing to conform to liberal ideologies of 'good mothering'.[2] Fundamental to these ideologies is the belief that 'good' mothers are self-disciplined and capable of meeting the needs of their families without assistance from the state (see also Anderson 2000; Kline 1993; Smith 1993). Specifically, exhortations that 'the health of the nation is the wealth of the nation' – which emerged in the classical liberal political milieu of 1920s and 1930s Canadian public-health messaging – took up ideals of maternal self-discipline and self-reliance by reifying women's obligations to support the state's economy by producing stronger (male) workers and soldiers (Arnup 1994). Contemporary neoliberal public-health messaging recapitulates these obligations, emphasizing women's responsibilities to have a 'healthy pregnancy' and a 'healthy baby' by avoiding alcohol, tobacco and other drugs. As funders of maternal education campaigns targeting FASD prevention, the state's primary interest is two-fold: first, to save tax dollars spent 'unnecessarily' on public services for children whose disabilities are 'entirely preventable'; and, second, to promote efforts that increase the availability of workers who will contribute to the national economy without becoming 'burdens' or 'drains' on the system.

These commitments are evident in many ways. When it comes to funding initiatives to prevent FASD, the Canadian government has, to date, allocated more resources to primary prevention campaigns than any other activity. In the western provinces and northern territories of Canada alone, over 350 separate FASD prevention campaigns have been launched in the past two decades (Thurmeir 2007). However, research strongly suggests that the women most likely to have a child with FASD are those least likely to be able to reduce their alcohol use on their own in response to public-health messages. In the most comprehensive study of birth mothers of children with foetal alcohol syndrome[3] conducted to date, Astley and colleagues (2000) found that all of the eighty women interviewed had addictions to alcohol that were intimately connected to extensive histories of severe physical, sexual and emotional abuse. In total, 80 per cent of the women interviewed were living with male partners who were violent and unsupportive of any efforts to quit drinking during their pregnancy. Most were socially isolated, living in poverty, with few supportive contacts with family members or friends. Most had also lost previous children to apprehension by child welfare authorities (see also Badry 2007; Salmon 2007a, 2007b). These findings have prompted concern amongst women's health researchers and service providers alike that primary prevention campaigns for FASD which increase knowledge about the harmful effects of foetal alcohol exposure without the supports needed by those women most likely to be drinking alcohol during pregnancy may inadvertently increase risks to maternal and child health by discouraging women from disclosing their substance use and pregnancies, and from seeking timely care (Boyd and Marcellus 2007; Salmon 2007a, 2007b; Tait 2000).

Early Canadian maternal education campaigns focused on producing healthy babies and children were initially confined to white, middle-class women, who had recently been removed from the paid labour force and were expected to focus their energies exclusively on mothering (Arnup 1994). Over time, the focus of these initiatives has shifted to emphasize the responsibility of Aboriginal, immigrant and impoverished mothers, among whose children rates of infant mortality, malnutrition and illness are highest. In practice, this shift has resulted in women from the poorest communities with the fewest resources gradually coming to shoulder the greatest burden for ensuring the health of their children. This dynamic remains evident in the contemporary positioning of Aboriginal women as targets for FASD prevention.

Through the administration of the Indian Act, First Nation, Inuit and Métis peoples remain formally disenfranchised in their relations with the Canadian state, and do not presently share all of the rights afforded to non-indigenous citizens in Canada. This results in the paradoxical positioning of Aboriginal mothers as having simultaneous duties to be both 'children of the state' and 'mothers of the nation' (Fiske 1993). The disenfranchisement of Aboriginal mothers as 'non-citizens' organizes the material conditions under which Aboriginal women in Canada live. To cite but one example, in 2009 Aboriginal children in the Canadian province of British Columbia were four-times more likely than non-Aboriginal children to have a child-protection concern reported, eight-times more likely to be found by child-welfare authorities to be in need of protection, and 5.6 times more likely to have their children apprehended and placed in foster care. Aboriginal children were also 12.3 times more likely to remain in foster care once apprehended (Ministry for Children and Family Development 2009). Swift (1995), Turpel (1993) and Fiske (1993) have observed that the over-representation of Aboriginal children in the child-welfare system is a direct result of the colonial legacy with which First Nations peoples in Canada live, including the residential schooling system.

This legacy is further mediated by positioning Aboriginal mothers as abusive, neglectful and otherwise dangerous to their children. Such constructions, coupled with increased opportunities for surveillance of Aboriginal women, families and communities enabled by government administrative practices, increases the likelihood that Aboriginal mothers will have their children removed from their care, particularly when they present for services disclosing that they have a substance-use problem (Fournier and Crey 1997; Royal Commission on Aboriginal Peoples 1996; Tait 2000; White and Jacobs 1992). Campaigns to prevent FASD must therefore be understood as emerging from a social, political and historical context in which Aboriginal mothers and their children have been repeatedly made objects of state intervention, including public-health interventions, and Aboriginal communities as sources of social problems that tax the resources of state institutions (Salmon 2004, 2007a, 2007b).

The role of alcohol in colonial and anti-colonial nation-building

Until 1951, Status Indians in BC (and other Canadian jurisdictions) were prohibited by law from drinking on reserve, and in public places off reserve. It was also illegal for anyone to sell or provide alcohol to an 'Indian'. Enforcing this colonial iteration of prohibition relied on finding ways to identify who could and could not consume alcohol, and under what conditions.[4] In this way, access to alcohol figured centrally in colonial constructions of 'the Indian' and of citizenship (Hamilton 2004).[5] Concerns about increasing legal access to alcohol were central in 1950s protests by indigenous leaders lobbying for changes to the Indian Act – not because First Nations, Inuit and Métis leaders were keen to increase alcohol consumption among Aboriginal people, but as a reaction to the paternalistic and segregationist value systems evident in the legislation that organized access to alcohol (Hamilton 2004).

Alcohol issues also figure predominantly in contemporary decolonization efforts in Canada. Arguing that the use of alcohol was not part of First Nations, Inuit and Métis societies prior to European contact, and that the introduction of alcohol has been intimately tied to conditions of colonization, some Aboriginal communities are becoming 'dry' as part of moves towards self-governance. Others are using their jurisdictional authority to initiate and enforce alcohol-control policies in which the commercial availability of alcohol is closely monitored and rationed, and drinking is prohibited among people with documented substance-use problems or who have exhibited destructive behaviour in connection to alcohol use (such as assaults or drink-driving). This approach is most commonly taken up in rural, remote and isolated communities.

Some indigenous leaders are also tying efforts to address problematic alcohol use to decolonization by articulating a view that high rates of substance use and related health problems (in some First Nation communities) are results of two interwoven experiences that mediate contemporary conditions of Aboriginal peoples and their communities (Thatcher 2004). The first is a recognition that high rates of alcohol use in some communities are the result of people's efforts to self-medicate against the effects of abuses suffered at government-sponsored and church-run residential schools (Milloy 1999; Thatcher 2004) and the legacy of the '60s scoop' – in which many Aboriginal children, usually the children and grandchildren of residential school survivors, were apprehended by child welfare authorities (Fournier and Crey 1997). The second is found in the view that high rates of problematic substance use are attributable to the current lack of social, economic, political and cultural opportunities for people (and particularly young people) on reserves and in rural and remote communities (Thatcher 2004). Here, it is argued that where basic services are scarce, unemployment rates are high, and where state interference has disrupted family and cultural systems that provided meaningful roles for community members, alcohol use becomes a default 'pastime' among those with few prospects for building a meaningful life for themselves and their families (Chandler and Lalonde 1998; Gagne 1998; Walters and Simoni 2002).

Situated in this context, alcohol use in pregnancy and the subsequent development of FASD can be seen as both a symptom and a legacy of the colonization of Indigenous peoples in Canada, and efforts to prevent it are the result of divergent, competing and sometimes contradictory discourses and ideologies. The following excerpt from *It Takes a Community* – a popular manual used to guide FASD-prevention efforts in indigenous communities – serves as an example of views of FASD prevention that are explicitly linked to an analysis of the impact of colonization:

Having been stripped of political agency on the nation level because of colonial attitudes of dominance and paternalism, First Nations and Inuit families and communities find themselves with decreased levels of self-sufficiency.... For instance, as a result of their upbringing in residential schools, generations of First Nations and Inuit have been unable to develop traditional knowledge and skills, including basic parenting skills. In the face of enduring these hardships and cultural disruption, addictions and substance abuse have become prevalent in Aboriginal communities.... Furthermore, an intergenerational cycle of physical, psychological, sexual abuse, and loss of spiritual practices, has sprung from this history of devaluation and control, providing fertile soil for addictions, alcoholism, and substance abuse.

(Van Bibber 1997: 4)

The incorporation of decolonization agendas into FASD-prevention campaigns targeting Aboriginal women and communities continues to be used as a strategy for accessing much-needed state resources. Linking public-health concerns to a decolonizing agenda has had success in bringing issues facing under-served women, children and families to the attention of state funders and policy-makers.

While this approach may have instrumental value in assisting communities to get programmes funded or to raise awareness of maternal and child health concerns, hegemonic understandings of what causes FASD and why it needs to be prevented remain intact: the targets for FASD-prevention messages are pregnant women who drink (not the state policies that perpetuate colonial conditions and health disparities), and 'FASD births' (i.e. Aboriginal children whose mothers drank during their gestation) need to be prevented because they represent extraordinary costs to communities and state institutions. To illustrate, in appealing to the 'extra lifetime costs' associated with foetal alcohol exposure, *It Takes a Community* argues for continued funding for FASD identification and 'risk reduction' programmes:

> the extra lifetime health care, education, corrections, and social services costs to society associated with an [FASD] individual have been estimated at US$1.4 million.... Since it [this estimate] is over 10 years old and applies to an American context, it is almost certainly an underestimate of the extra lifetime costs associated with caring for an FAS individual in Canada.
>
> This estimate illustrates the potential costs that FASD represents. Take the extra lifetime costs per FAS-affected individual (US$1.4 million) and multiply it by the incidence of FAS (potentially 740 FAS births a year in Canada). The total is over US$1 billion; this represents the total cost (in monetary terms alone) of FAS to Canadian society for one birth cohort alone.... This cost needs to be balanced against the continuing annual funding allocated to the [First Nations and Inuit FAS/FAE[6] Prevention] Initiative (CND$1.7 million) when making FAS/FAE funding decisions in the future.
>
> (Van Bibber 1997: 23)

This statement demonstrates the influence of neoliberalist ideologies on FASD-prevention initiatives. Although they have instrumental value as tools for garnering political support for preventative initiatives, using economic costing arguments can also undermine social justice by suggesting that Aboriginal mothers who give birth to children with FASD threaten the interests of state institutions, in the form of the 'extra lifetime costs' they pose to those (presumably limited) resources. As a result, they are positioned as legitimate targets of public-health interventions to modify their behaviour and, in some cases, infringe upon their reproductive autonomy (Tait 2000). Moreover, it is suggested that these 'extra lifetime costs' cannot be met, nor should they be expected to be met, through state resources. Given the neoliberalist orientation of the contemporary Canadian welfare state, the needs and interests (and indeed the existence) of persons with FASD are therefore seen as being at odds with the needs, interests and expectations of 'Canadian society'.

FASD prevention and the contestations of neoliberalist and decolonizing agendas

As Tait (2000: 104) has noted:

> FAS research, population assessments and prevention programs in Canada have been located in First Nation communities since alcohol abuse has been identified by many First Nation communities as one of the major health problems confronting them. This has meant that health issues related to substance abuse, such as addiction treatment, and prevention of FAS have been prioritized by communities themselves.

First Nation, Inuit, and Métis peoples in Canada have indeed shown tremendous leadership in taking on FASD prevention as a priority area for public-health action at the community and national levels, and in advancing holistic, integrated approaches to FASD prevention that extend beyond reductivist, individualized 'shame and blame' foci evident in much mainstream public-health work (Salmon 2004). Nonetheless, while preventing FASD is an important public-health and social-justice aspiration, it must also be acknowledged that FASD prevention can also feed into neoliberal policy agendas in ways that can compromise social-justice concerns of Aboriginal peoples, women and people with disabilities.

Shifts towards neoliberal policy agendas over the past two decades have placed demands on nations to create 'lean-states' by restructuring social programmes. These moves favour initiatives that devolve responsibilities – including shifting responsibilities for ensuring the health and well-being of marginalized peoples from the state to community-based or private organizations. They also favour interventions to decrease individual 'dependency' on or costs to the state. These trends have informed political decisions to fund FASD initiatives that rely on Aboriginal communities (rather than the state) to undertake prevention efforts on the grounds that 'FASD births' represent an 'entirely preventable' and unjustifiable 'cost to communities'. Critical examination of some of the more problematic undercurrents in FASD-prevention initiatives thus demands an analysis of how neoliberalist, anti-colonial and public-health agendas are enacted by the state (directly and indirectly) on the bodies of Aboriginal women and their children in ways that may be problematic for advancing their health, well-being and citizenship interests.

In Western neoliberal policy contexts, articulations of citizenship are grounded in an assumed ability to participate in activities that produce sufficient economic value to support an individual's needs, the needs of his or her 'dependents' and the needs of national economies (Stone 1984). In the relevancies of neoliberal politics, 'good citizens' are good workers who contribute monetary wealth to local and national economics while placing few (if any) demands on state resources. Thus, productivist constructions of citizenship can remove people with disabilities, Aboriginal peoples and women from capitalist circuits of production by representing them as 'burdens', 'drains' or even 'threats' to the institutions and economies of the nation-state (Meekosha 1999; Meekosha and Dowse 1997). By placing them outside these circuits, ideologies of 'productive citizenship' thus also deny these groups much of their entitlement to consideration as 'citizens'. At the same time, this discourse obscures the structural and institutional factors that differentially enable some individuals and groups to participate in communities, economies and institutions as 'citizens' (Salmon 2007b). Women who give birth to children with disabilities are often constructed as 'failing' both tests of citizenship: they are seen to have 'produced' children who are 'burdens' on already over-taxed health, education, social service and (in the case of FASD) criminal-legal systems. Moreover, due to the extraordinary care-giving responsibilities faced by mothers of disabled children in the absence of a strong system of public services, such mothers often remove themselves (often involuntarily) from paid work, often with little recourse but to go on social assistance in an attempt to meet their families' basic needs. This is turn provides a vehicle through which policy-makers can mobilize discursively mediated practices that position the 'needs' of poor, racialized women and their children against those of 'the public' in an attempt to secure public consent for the dismantling or implementation of specific social programmes.

While critically important for Aboriginal peoples, decolonization movements aiming to achieve social, cultural, political and economic justice can also feed into neoliberal agendas to create 'leaner states'. Put bluntly, devolving responsibilities for governance and service provision from federal, provincial and territorial governments onto First Nation, Inuit and Métis governments can save the state money and remove its accountability for ensuring the rights and well-being of indigenous peoples (for further discussion of this topic, see Irlbacher-Fox 2009). Some First Nation leaders, including senior health administrators, have criticized the Canadian government for negotiating settlements with indigenous peoples that increase their responsibility to provide services without the accompanying resources required to ensure the care their communities need (Sommerfeld and Payne 2004). This has occurred most recently in First Nation communities in the delegation of authority for child-welfare agencies, housing and water quality on reserves, and is now increasingly evident in other aspects of public health (Sommerfeld and Payne 2004). Some commentators have further noted that these crises for indigenous communities – that result from devolution of responsibility for governance and service provision to First Nation governments without adequate resources to meet these obligations – can create situations that play to racist tropes and constructions of Aboriginal peoples as unable to care for themselves, giving rise to 'an image of sick, disorganized communities [which] can be used to justify paternalism and dependency' (O'Neil 1993: 34).

Conclusion

Linking FASD prevention to decolonization efforts in the context of a neoliberal policy environment demands caution. On the one hand, the neoliberalist impulse can assist communities in securing funding for prevention campaigns, using the rationale that FASD prevention saves public money. As I have argued, this is often seen in the strategic deployment of statistics related to the 'lifetime cost' a person with FASD imposes on government institutions. Thus, the operationalization of neoliberal ideologies can create conditions in which some innovative FASD-prevention campaigns tied to decolonization are funded, allowing the concerns of disenfranchised peoples to be addressed through the state. In this sense, as Martell (2000: 212) notes, FASD prevention can provide opportunities for 'collective power in community development', underscoring 'the importance of honouring each community's unique cultural and community spirit in finding their own answers [to FASD]'. Consequently, 'moral discourse [surrounding FASD prevention] identifies a concrete problem around which organizations can lobby for scarce, but badly needed, government funding' (Tait 2000: 103).

One the other hand, FASD is a condition unparalleled in its complexity as both a public-health issue and an expression of disenfranchisement and abandonment. Its prevention requires comprehensive responses to support change that can rarely be measured over the short term in which brief windows of policy attention are typically offered. When community leaders argue for access to funds for programmes to prevent FASD – at moments in time when the local incidence and prevalence of the condition may not be concretely known, and where gains made in 'high-risk' women's health and well-being are likely to be achieved incrementally over many years –

those leaders risk being blamed for 'failure' if progress cannot be definitively documented and shown in a short period of time. This is the situation confronting most FASD-prevention programmes in Canada – indigenous or otherwise – and it is a shaky foundation on which to build and improve services for women, children and families facing severe disadvantage (Tait 2008). This raises important questions for indigenous peoples, service providers and policy-makers. When FASD prevention as a public-health goal is linked to decolonization but articulated through the relevancies of neoliberal ideologies, who benefits? What political agendas are progressed and on what terms? And what are the consequences for Aboriginal mothers, their children and their communities?

Notes

Acknowledgements: I would like to thank Marilyn Van Bibber for generously sharing insights that have shaped my thinking on the issues discussed in this chapter.

1 For a discussion of the politics of 'counting' in public-health surveillance research, see Mair (this volume).
2 For discussions related to interventions to address childhood obesity, see McNaughton's and LeBesco's chapters in this volume.
3 Foetal alcohol syndrome is one type of FASD, characterized by specific facial features, low birth weight and slow postnatal growth, organ damage, cognitive impairment and developmental delay.
4 Similar patterns in Aboriginal alcohol policy are evident in Australia. For a complete discussion of alcohol policy in relation to Aboriginal communities in Australia, see Brady 2004.
5 Prior to the 1950s, 'Indians' could only drink alcohol legally if they became 'enfranchised', formally giving up their treaty rights (or, in the absence of treaties, rights guaranteed under the Indian Act).
6 FAE is an abbreviation for 'foetal alcohol effects', a descriptive term used prior to the adoption of the term FASD.

References

Adlaf, E.M., Begin, P. and Sawka, E. (eds) (2005) *Canadian Addictions Survey (CAS): A National Survey of Canadians' Use of Alcohol and Other Drugs*, Ottawa: Canadian Centre on Substance Abuse.

Anderson, K. (2000) *A Recognition of Being: Reconstructing Native Womanhood*, Toronto: Second Story Press.

Armstrong, E.M. (2003) *Conceiving Risk, Bearing Responsibility: Fetal Alcohol Syndrome and the Diagnosis of Moral Disorder*, Baltimore and London: John Hopkins University Press.

Arnup, K. (1994) *Education for Motherhood: Advice for Mothers in Twentieth-Century Canada*, Toronto: University of Toronto Press.

Asante, K.O. and Nelms-Matzke, J. (1985) *Survey of Children With Chronic Handicaps and Fetal Alcohol Syndrome in the Yukon and Northwest of British Columbia*, Ottawa: Health and Welfare Canada.

Astley, S., Bailey, D., Talbot, C. and Clarren, S. (2000) 'Fetal Alcohol Syndrome primary prevention through diagnosis: I. Identification of high risk birth mothers through the diagnosis of their children and II. A comprehensive profile of 80 birth mothers of children with FAS', *Alcohol*, 35(5): 499–519.

Badry, D. (2007) 'Birth mothers of children with fetal alcohol syndrome', in M.J. Jackson, M.J. Pickard and E.W. Bawner (eds) *Social Justice in Context*, vol. 3 2007–2008, Greenville: Carolyn Freeze Baynes Institute for Social Justice, pp. 88–108.

Bollin, K., Grant, C., Hamlyn, B. and Thornton, A. (2007) *Infant Feeding Survey 2005*, Leeds: The Information Centre.

Boyd, S.C. and Marcellus, L. (eds) (2007) *With Child: Substance Use During Pregnancy – A Woman-Centred Approach*, Vancouver: Fernwood Publishing.

Brady, M. (2004) *Indigenous Australia and Alcohol Policy: Meeting Difference with Indifference*, Sydney: University of New South Wales Press.

British Medical Association (2007) *Fetal Alcohol Spectrum Disorders*, London: BMA.

Centers for Disease Control (2002) 'FAS: Alaska, Arizona, Colorado, and New York 1995–1997', *Morbidity and Mortality Weekly Report*, 514: 433–435.

Chandler, J.J. and Lalonde, C. (1998) 'Cultural continuity as a hedge against suicide in Canada's First Nations', *Transcultural Psychiatry*, 35(5): 191–219.

Clarren, S. and Smith, D.W. (1978) 'The fetal alcohol syndrome', *New England Journal of Medicine*, 298(19): 1063–1067.

Colvin, L., Payne, J., Parsons, D., Kurinczuk, J. and Bower, C. (2007) 'Alcohol consumption during pregnant in nonindigenous western Australian women', *Alcoholism: Clinical and Experimental Research*, 31(2): 276–284.

Environics Research Group (2006) *Alcohol Use During Pregnancy and Awareness of Fetal Alcohol Syndrome and Fetal Alcohol Spectrum Disorder: Results of a National Survey*, Ottawa: Public Health Agency of Canada.

Fiske, J. (1993) 'Child of the state, mother of the nation: Aboriginal women and the ideology of motherhood', *Culture*, 1(3): 17–35.

Floyd, R.L., Sobell, M., Valasques, M.M., Ingersoll, K., Nettleman, M., Sobell, L., Mullan, P.D., Ceperich, S., von Sternberg, K., Bolton, B., Skarpness, B. and Nagaraja, J. (2007) 'Preventing alcohol exposed pregnancies: A randomized controlled trial', *American Journal of Preventive Medicine*, 32(1): 1–10.

Fournier, S. and Crey, E. (1997) *Stolen From our Embrace: The Abduction of First Nations Children and the Restoration of Aboriginal Communities*, Vancouver: Douglas and McIntyre.

Gagne, M. (1998) 'The role of dependency and colonialism in generating trauma in First Nations citizens', in Y. Danieli (ed.) *International Handbook of Multigenerational Legacies of Trauma*, New York: Plenium Press, pp. 355–372.

Hamilton, D.L. (2004) *Sobering Dilemma: A History of Prohibition in British Columbia*, Vancouver: Ronsdale Press.

Health Canada (1996) *Joint Statement: Prevention of Fetal Alcohol Syndrome (FASD) and Fetal Alcohol Effects (FAE)*, Ottawa: Health Canada.

Irlbacher-Fox, S. (2009) *Finding Dahshaa: Self Government, Social Suffering, and Aboriginal Policy in Canada*, Vancouver: University of British Columbia Press.

Kline, M. (1993) 'Complicating the ideology of motherhood: Child welfare law and First Nations women', *Queen's Law Journal*, 15(2): 306–342.

Maier, S.E. and West, J.R. (2001) 'Drinking patterns and alcohol related birth defects', *Alcohol Research and Health*, 25(3): 168–174F.

Martell, R. (2002) 'Fetal Alcohol Syndrome: The Teachers Among Us', in K. Anderson and B. Lawrence (eds) *Strong Women Stories: Native Vision and Community Survival*, Toronto: Sumach Press, pp. 202–212.

May, P.A., Gossage, J.P., White-Country, M., Goodhart, K., Decoteau, S., Trujillo, P.M., Kalberg, W.O., Viljoen, D.L. and Hoyme, H.E. (2004) 'Alcohol consumption and other maternal risk factors for fetal alcohol syndrome among three distinct samples of women before, during, and after pregnancy: The risk is relative', *American Journal of Medical Genetics*, 127C(1): 10–20.

Meekosha, H. (1999) 'Disability, political activism, and identity making: A critical feminist perspective on the rise of disability movements in Australia, the USA, and the UK', *Disability Studies Quarterly*, 19(4): n.p.

Meekosha, H. and Dowse, L. (1997) 'Enabling citizenship: Gender, disability, and citizenship', *Feminist Review*, Autumn: 49–72.

Milloy, J.S. (1999) *A National Crime: The Canadian Government and the Residential School System*, Winnipeg: University of Manitoba Press.

Ministry for Children and Family Development (2009) *Aboriginal Children in Care*, Victoria: MCFD Research, Analysis, and Evaluation Branch.

O'Neil, J.D. (1993) *Aboriginal Health Policy For the Next Century. Report of the Royal Commission on Aboriginal Peoples: The Path of Healing*, Ottawa: Minister of Supply and Services Canada.

Poole, N. and Dell, C.A. (2005) *Girls, Women, and Substance Use*, Ottawa and Vancouver: Canadian Centre on Substance Abuse and BC Centre of Excellence for Women's Health.

Robinson, G.C., Conry, J.L. and Conry, R.F. (1987) 'Clinical profile and prevalence of fetal alcohol syndrome in an isolated community in British Columbia', *Canadian Medical Association Journal*, 137(3): 203–207.

Royal Australian and New Zealand College of Obstetricians and Gynaecologists (2008) *College Statement: Alcohol in Pregnancy*, East Melbourne: RANWCOG.

Royal College of Obstetricians and Gynaecologists (2006) *RCOG Statement No. 5: Alcohol Consumption and the Outcomes of Pregnancy*, London: RCOG.

Royal Commission on Aboriginal Peoples (1996) *Report of the Royal Commission on Aboriginal Peoples*, Ottawa: Minister of Supply and Services Canada.

Salmon, A. (2004) ' "It takes a community": constructing Aboriginal mothers and children with FAS/FAE as objects of moral panic in/through a FAS/FAE prevention policy', *Journal of the Association for Research on Mothering*, 6(1): 112–123.

Salmon, A. (2007a) 'Adaptation and decolonization: The role of "culturally appropriate" health education in the prevention of fetal alcohol syndrome', *Canadian Journal of Native Education*, 30(2): 257–274.

Salmon, A. (2007b) 'Dis/abling states, dis/abling citizenship: Young Aboriginal mothers, substantive citizenship, and the medicalization of FAS/FAE', *Journal of Critical Education Policy*, 5(2): 112–123.

Smith, D.E. (1993) 'The standard North American family: SNAF as ideological code', *Journal of Family Issues*, 14(1): 50–65.

Sommerfeld, M. and Payne, H. (2004) *Entrenched Incapacity and the Rights of Small Independent First Nations in the Delivery of Community Health Services*, Nanaimo: Intertribal Health Authority.

Stone, D. (1984) *The Disabled State*, Philadelphia: Temple University Press.

Swift, K. (1995) *Manufacturing Bad Mothers: A Critical Perspective on Child Neglect*, Toronto: University of Toronto Press.

Tait, C.L. (2000) *A Study of the Service Needs of Pregnant Addicted Women in Manitoba*, Winnipeg: Manitoba Health.

Tait, C.L. (2003) *Fetal Alcohol Syndrome Among Canadian Aboriginal Peoples: Review and Analysis of the Intergenerational Links to Residential Schools*, Ottawa: The Aboriginal Healing Foundation.

Tait, C.L. (2008) 'Ethical programming: Toward a community-centred approach to mental health and addiction programming in Aboriginal communities', *Pimatisiwin: A Journal of Aboriginal and Community Health*, 6(1): 29–60.

Thatcher, R.W. (2004) *Fighting Firewater Fictions: Moving Beyond the Disease Model of Alcoholism in First Nations*, Toronto: University of Toronto Press.

Thurmeir, R. (2007) *Creating Effective Primary Prevention FASD Resources: Evaluation Processes in Health Promotion*, Saskatoon: Saskatchewan Prevention Institute.

Turpel, M. (1993) 'Patriarchy and paternalism: The legacy of the Canadian state for First Nations women', *Canadian Journal of Women and the Law*, 6(1): 174–192.

US Surgeon General (2005) *Surgeon General's Advisory on Alcohol Use in Pregnancy*, Washington, DC: Office of the US Surgeon General.

Van Bibber, M. (1997) *It Takes a Community: A Resource Manual for Community-Based Prevention of FAS and FAE*, Ottawa: Health Canada.

Walters, K.L. and Simoni, J.M. (2002) 'Reconceptualizing native women's health: An "indigenist" stress-coping model', *American Journal of Public Health*, 92(4): 520–524.

White, L. and Jacobs, E. (1992) *Liberating our Children, Liberating our Nations: Report of the Aboriginal Committee Community Panel, Family and Children's Services Legislation Review in British Columbia*, Victoria, BC: The Committee.

Index

Note: Page numbers in **bold** denote figures, those in *italics* denote tables.

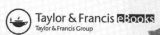

Printed and bound by CPI Group (UK) Ltd, Croydon, CR0 4YY

01/11/2024

01782630-0015